CARB CYCLING FOR WOMEN OVER 50

Achieving Wellness: Carb Management Tactics for Seniors
Beyond Fifty

Sophia j. Smith

INTRODUCTION

Welcome to "Carb Cycling for Women Over 50," your comprehensive guide to optimizing health, vitality, and fitness through a tailored approach to nutrition. As we navigate the unique challenges and opportunities that come with age, finding effective strategies for maintaining a healthy weight, boosting energy levels, and supporting overall well-being becomes increasingly important.

Carb cycling offers a dynamic and flexible way to achieve these goals by strategically alternating between high and low-carbohydrate intake days. This method not only supports metabolic efficiency but also aligns with the evolving nutritional needs of women over 50, promoting sustainable weight management and enhancing performance in daily activities and fitness routines.

In this book, we delve into the science behind carb cycling, exploring how this approach can positively impact metabolism, hormone balance, and overall health. You will gain insights into why carb cycling is particularly beneficial for women in their 50s and beyond, providing a pathway to maintaining muscle mass, managing weight fluctuations, and optimizing energy levels.

We guide you through the practical implementation of carb cycling, offering personalized strategies and meal plans designed to fit seamlessly into your lifestyle. From understanding macronutrient needs to crafting delicious and nutritious recipes, each chapter is crafted to empower you with the knowledge and tools necessary to thrive on your health journey.

Beyond nutrition, we address the holistic aspects of well-being essential for women over 50. From incorporating suitable exercise routines and stress management techniques to enhancing sleep quality and overall mental resilience, this book equips you with a comprehensive approach to living vibrantly and healthily.

Whether you are new to carb cycling or looking to refine your approach, "Carb Cycling for Women Over 50" serves as your trusted companion. Embrace this journey with enthusiasm and determination, knowing that each step you take towards optimizing your health is a step towards a more fulfilling and active life.

TABLE OF CONTENTS

Chapter 1: Welcome

1.1 What is Carb Cycling?

Carb cycling is a dietary strategy that involves alternating between periods of higher and lower carbohydrate intake. Rather than consistently consuming the same amount of carbs every day, carb cycling varies carbohydrate consumption based on specific goals, such as athletic performance, fat loss, or muscle gain.

How Carb Cycling Works:
1. High-Carb Days:

- These days involve consuming a higher amount of carbohydrates, typically focusing on complex carbs like whole grains, vegetables, and fruits.
- High-carb days are often scheduled around intense physical activity or workouts to provide ample energy for performance and recovery.
- The increased carb intake can replenish glycogen stores in muscles, supporting endurance and preventing fatigue.

2. Low-Carb Days:

- On low-carb days, carbohydrate intake is reduced, emphasizing lean proteins, healthy fats, and non-starchy vegetables.
- This phase aims to promote fat burning by forcing the body to rely more on stored fat for energy, a process known as ketosis in extreme low-carb diets.
- Low-carb days also help stabilize blood sugar levels and insulin response, which can aid in weight management and metabolic health.

1.2 Why Carb Cycling for Women Over 50?

Carb cycling holds significant benefits for women over 50, addressing specific physiological changes and health considerations that come with age. Here's why carb cycling can be particularly advantageous for this demographic:

1. Metabolic Support and Hormonal Balance
Hormonal Changes: Women over 50 often experience hormonal shifts, particularly during menopause. Carb cycling can help manage insulin levels and support hormonal balance, which is crucial for maintaining metabolism and energy levels.

Metabolic Flexibility: As metabolism naturally slows with age, carb cycling promotes metabolic flexibility by alternating between high and low carb days. This approach can help prevent metabolic adaptation to low-calorie diets, aiding in weight management.

2. Weight Management and Body Composition
Preserving Lean Muscle: Carb cycling supports muscle maintenance and growth, which is essential for women over 50 to counteract age-related muscle loss (sarcopenia).

Fat Loss: Alternating carb intake can optimize fat loss by promoting the use of stored fat as energy during low-carb days, while high-carb days replenish glycogen stores for energy and performance.

3. Energy Levels and Physical Performance
Sustained Energy: By strategically timing carbohydrate intake, women over 50 can maintain consistent energy levels throughout the day. High-carb days provide fuel for physical activities and exercise, while low-carb days encourage fat utilization for prolonged energy.

4. Blood Sugar Management and Insulin Sensitivity

Stable Blood Sugar: Carb cycling helps stabilize blood sugar levels, reducing the risk of insulin resistance and promoting better glucose control. This is particularly beneficial for women over 50 who may be at higher risk of metabolic disorders.

5. Adaptability to Lifestyle and Preferences

Flexibility: Carb cycling offers a flexible approach to nutrition, allowing for adjustments based on individual preferences, activity levels, and health goals.

Sustainability: It can be adapted to accommodate dietary preferences such as vegetarianism or gluten-free diets, making it easier for women over 50 to maintain long-term adherence.

6. Overall Health Benefits

Heart Health: A balanced approach to carb cycling, focusing on whole grains, fruits, and vegetables, supports heart health by reducing cholesterol levels and promoting cardiovascular function.

Mental Clarity and Mood: Stable blood sugar levels from carb cycling can enhance cognitive function and mood stability, contributing to overall well-being.

Carb cycling for women over 50 offers a tailored approach to nutrition that addresses age-related changes while promoting overall health, vitality, and longevity. By incorporating this strategy into their lifestyle, women in this demographic can optimize their metabolic health, manage weight effectively, and maintain energy levels for a vibrant and active life.

Chapter 2: Understanding Carb Cycling

2.1 The Science Behind Carb Cycling

Carb cycling is rooted in metabolic science and the physiological responses of the body to varying levels of carbohydrate intake. Understanding the science behind carb cycling can shed light on why this dietary strategy is effective for many individuals seeking to manage weight, optimize performance, and improve metabolic health.

Metabolic Adaptation

Carbohydrate Utilization: Carbohydrates are the body's primary source of energy, particularly for high-intensity activities and brain function. When consumed, carbohydrates are broken down into glucose, which fuels cells throughout the body.

Insulin Response: Carbohydrate intake triggers the release of insulin, a hormone that helps transport glucose into cells for energy or storage. Excessive carb consumption can lead to insulin resistance over time, impacting metabolic health.

The Role of Glycogen

Glycogen Stores: Excess glucose not immediately used for energy is stored in the muscles and liver as glycogen. Glycogen serves as a readily available energy reserve that can be tapped into during physical activity or periods of reduced carbohydrate intake.

Glycogen Depletion: During low-carb phases of carb cycling, glycogen stores are gradually depleted. This prompts the body to rely more on stored fat for energy, leading to increased fat burning and potentially facilitating weight loss.

Hormonal and Metabolic Adaptation

Hormonal Balance: Carb cycling helps regulate insulin levels, which in turn influences other hormones involved in metabolism and appetite regulation. By alternating between high and low carb days, insulin sensitivity can be improved, supporting overall metabolic health.

Adaptation to Change: The body adapts to changes in carbohydrate intake by adjusting its metabolic pathways. High-carb days stimulate glycogen replenishment and support muscle recovery and growth, while low-carb days encourage fat utilization and metabolic flexibility.

Performance and Recovery

Athletic Performance: Timing carbohydrate intake around workouts can enhance performance by providing the necessary energy for endurance and strength training activities. High-carb days ensure adequate glycogen stores for optimal physical performance.

Recovery: Post-exercise, carbohydrates aid in muscle glycogen restoration and recovery. Carb cycling allows for strategic replenishment of glycogen stores while promoting fat utilization during rest days or lower activity periods.

Individual Variation and Adaptability

Personalized Approach: Carb cycling can be customized based on individual goals, activity levels, and metabolic needs. This flexibility makes it suitable for a wide range of individuals, from athletes seeking performance gains to individuals managing weight or metabolic conditions.

Understanding the science behind carb cycling highlights its effectiveness in optimizing energy metabolism, promoting fat loss, and supporting overall metabolic health. By strategically alternating between periods of high and low carbohydrate intake, individuals can harness the benefits of both energy efficiency and fat utilization, tailored to their specific health and fitness goals.

2.2 Benefits of Carb Cycling

Carb cycling offers a variety of benefits that make it a popular dietary strategy among individuals aiming to optimize their health, manage weight, and enhance athletic performance. Here are some key advantages of carb cycling:

1. Enhanced Fat Loss
Metabolic Flexibility: Alternating between high and low carb days encourages the body to switch between using carbohydrates and fats for energy. Low-carb days promote fat burning, helping to reduce body fat percentage over time.

Preservation of Lean Muscle: Unlike traditional low-calorie diets that may lead to muscle loss, carb cycling supports muscle preservation. High-carb days provide adequate energy for workouts, while low-carb days promote fat utilization without sacrificing muscle mass.

2. Improved Metabolic Health
Insulin Sensitivity: Carb cycling can improve insulin sensitivity, reducing the risk of insulin resistance and type 2 diabetes. Alternating carbohydrate intake helps regulate blood sugar levels and prevents spikes in insulin, promoting better metabolic health.

Stable Energy Levels: By managing glycogen stores effectively, carb cycling helps maintain consistent energy levels throughout the day. This is particularly beneficial for athletes and individuals with demanding lifestyles.

3. Optimized Athletic Performance
Fuel for Workouts: High-carb days provide sufficient glycogen stores to fuel intense workouts and enhance athletic performance. Carbohydrates are crucial for high-intensity exercise, supporting endurance and recovery.

Adaptation to Training: Carb cycling allows athletes to adapt their carbohydrate intake to match training demands. This strategic approach can improve training outcomes and recovery, leading to better overall performance.

4. Flexible and Sustainable

Adaptability: Carb cycling can be tailored to individual preferences, dietary needs, and fitness goals. It offers flexibility in food choices and meal planning, making it easier to adhere to long-term compared to strict dietary regimens.

Psychological Benefits: The variety provided by carb cycling prevents monotony and deprivation often associated with traditional diets. This can improve adherence and reduce cravings, supporting sustainable lifestyle changes.

5. Supports Hormonal Balance

Women's Health: For women, carb cycling can help regulate hormones involved in metabolism and reproductive health. It may be particularly beneficial during phases of hormonal fluctuation such as menopause, promoting weight management and overall well-being.

6. Potential Health Benefits

Heart Health: Balanced carb cycling plans that emphasize whole grains, fruits, and vegetables can support heart health by reducing cholesterol levels and promoting cardiovascular function.

Mental Clarity: Stable blood sugar levels from carb cycling can enhance cognitive function and mood stability, contributing to overall mental well-being.

Carb cycling offers a scientifically grounded approach to nutrition that balances energy needs, promotes fat loss, and supports metabolic health. By strategically alternating between high and low carbohydrate intake, individuals can achieve their health and fitness goals while enjoying the flexibility and sustainability of this dietary strategy. Whether aiming for weight loss, athletic performance enhancement, or improved metabolic function, carb cycling provides a versatile tool for optimizing overall health and well-being.

2.3 Carb Cycling vs. Other Diets

Carb cycling stands out among various dietary approaches due to its unique method of alternating carbohydrate intake. Here's how carb cycling compares to other popular diets:

1. Low-Carb Diets (e.g., Keto Diet)

Carb Restriction: Low-carb diets like keto drastically reduce carbohydrate intake to induce ketosis, a metabolic state where the body burns fat for fuel.

Focus: Keto diets focus on high fat intake, moderate protein consumption, and very low carbohydrate intake (typically less than 50 grams per day).

Purpose: Keto aims for sustained ketosis to maximize fat burning, weight loss, and metabolic benefits.

2. High-Carb Diets

Standard Approach: Traditional high-carb diets emphasize ample carbohydrate intake for energy, often including grains, fruits, and starchy vegetables.

Purpose: Suitable for athletes or those with high energy needs, emphasizing performance and glycogen replenishment.

Considerations: High-carb diets may lead to insulin spikes, energy crashes, and potential weight gain if calorie intake exceeds energy expenditure.

3. Intermittent Fasting

Time-Restricted Eating: Intermittent fasting alternates between periods of eating and fasting, such as the 16/8 method (16 hours fasting, 8 hours eating window).

Purpose: Focuses on timing of meals rather than specific macronutrient ratios. May enhance fat burning, improve insulin sensitivity, and support metabolic health.

Flexibility: Allows for varied eating patterns, potentially improving adherence and promoting sustainable weight management.

4. Calorie Restriction Diets

Reduced Caloric Intake: Calorie restriction involves consuming fewer calories than expended, promoting weight loss by creating a calorie deficit.

Focus: Primarily on total energy balance rather than macronutrient composition. May lead to weight loss but can also result in muscle loss if not combined with adequate protein intake and exercise.

Long-term Sustainability: May be challenging to sustain due to feelings of deprivation and potential metabolic adaptations.

5. Paleo Diet

Whole Foods Approach: The Paleo diet emphasizes whole, unprocessed foods similar to those available to our ancestors during the Paleolithic era.

Focus: Includes lean proteins, fruits, vegetables, nuts, and seeds while excluding grains, dairy, and processed foods.

Purpose: Supports overall health by focusing on nutrient-dense foods and avoiding processed ingredients, but does not specifically regulate carbohydrate intake.

6. Mediterranean Diet

Heart-Healthy Approach: The Mediterranean diet emphasizes fruits, vegetables, whole grains, legumes, and healthy fats like olive oil and nuts.

Focus: Promotes cardiovascular health, reducing the risk of heart disease and improving overall well-being.

Moderate Carbohydrates: Includes moderate carbohydrate intake primarily from whole grains and legumes, but does not manipulate carb intake for specific metabolic benefits.

Carb cycling differs from other diets by strategically alternating carbohydrate intake to optimize metabolic responses, support fat loss, and enhance performance. Unlike strict low-carb or high-carb diets, carb cycling offers flexibility, adapts to individual needs, and can be customized based on goals, activity levels, and metabolic health. By balancing carbohydrate intake with periods of lower consumption, carb cycling provides a versatile approach to nutrition that can be sustainable and effective for achieving long-term health and fitness goals.

Chapter 3: Nutrition Basics

3.1 Macronutrients: Carbs, Proteins, and Fats

Understanding macronutrients—carbohydrates, proteins, and fats—is essential for implementing an effective carb cycling plan. Each macronutrient plays a unique role in the body's energy metabolism, muscle function, and overall health.

Carbohydrates

- Role: Carbohydrates are the body's primary source of energy. They are broken down into glucose, which fuels cells, particularly the brain and muscles.
- Types: Carbs are classified as simple (sugars) or complex (starches and fibers). Complex carbs provide sustained energy and are found in whole grains, fruits, vegetables, and legumes.
- Carb Cycling Strategy: During high-carb days, focus on whole grains, fruits, and vegetables to replenish glycogen stores and fuel intense workouts. On low-carb days, limit carbs to promote fat burning and stabilize blood sugar levels.

Proteins

- Role: Proteins are essential for building and repairing tissues, including muscles, bones, skin, and enzymes. They also play a role in hormone regulation and immune function.
- Sources: Proteins are found in meat, poultry, fish, eggs, dairy products, legumes, nuts, and seeds.
- Carb Cycling Strategy: Consume adequate protein to support muscle maintenance and growth. Protein intake should be consistent throughout carb cycling phases to prevent muscle loss during low-carb periods.

Fats

- Role: Fats are a concentrated source of energy and are vital for cell structure, hormone production, and nutrient absorption (such as fat-soluble vitamins A, D, E, and K).
- Types: Healthy fats include monounsaturated and polyunsaturated fats found in olive oil, avocados, nuts, and fatty fish. Saturated fats, found in animal products and some plant oils, should be consumed in moderation.
- Carb Cycling Strategy: Include healthy fats in each meal to support satiety and nutrient absorption. During low-carb days, prioritize fats as an alternative energy source, promoting ketosis and fat metabolism.

Balancing Macronutrients in Carb Cycling

- High-Carb Days: Emphasize complex carbohydrates to fuel workouts and replenish glycogen stores. Include lean proteins and moderate fats to support muscle recovery and overall energy balance.

- Low-Carb Days: Focus on lean proteins, healthy fats, and non-starchy vegetables to promote fat burning and stabilize blood sugar levels. Limit carbohydrate intake to facilitate ketosis and enhance metabolic flexibility.

Macronutrients—carbohydrates, proteins, and fats—play crucial roles in supporting overall health and optimizing performance during carb cycling. By strategically adjusting macronutrient intake based on daily activity levels and goals, individuals can achieve sustainable weight management, enhance athletic performance, and promote metabolic health effectively. Balancing these nutrients ensures that each phase of carb cycling contributes to long-term well-being and fitness success.

3.2 Micronutrients: Vitamins and Minerals

Micronutrients, including vitamins and minerals, are essential for various physiological functions, metabolism, and overall health. While macronutrients (carbohydrates, proteins, fats) provide energy, micronutrients play critical roles as cofactors in enzymatic reactions, antioxidants, and regulators of cellular processes.

Vitamins

Fat-Soluble Vitamins:

- Vitamin A: Upholds vision, resistant capability, and skin wellbeing. Found in orange and yellow fruits, leafy greens, and dairy products.
- Vitamin D: Regulates calcium absorption, supporting bone health and immune function. Synthesized by the skin with sunlight exposure and found in fatty fish and fortified foods.
- Vitamin E: Goes about as a cancer prevention agent, shielding cells from harm. Found in nuts, seeds, and vegetable oils.
- Vitamin K: Fundamental for blood thickening and bone wellbeing. Found in leafy greens, broccoli, and vegetable oils.

Water-Soluble Vitamins:

- Vitamin B Complex: Includes B1 (thiamine), B2 (riboflavin), B3 (niacin), B5 (pantothenic acid), B6 (pyridoxine), B7 (biotin), B9 (folate), and B12 (cobalamin). These vitamins play roles in energy metabolism, nerve function, red blood cell formation, and DNA synthesis. Found in various foods, including whole grains, meat, fish, dairy, and leafy greens.
- Vitamin C: Acts as an antioxidant, supporting immune function, collagen synthesis, and iron absorption. Found in citrus natural products, berries, ringer peppers, and mixed greens.

Minerals

Macrominerals:

- Calcium: Fundamental for bone and teeth wellbeing, muscle capability, and nerve transmission. Found in dairy products, leafy greens, and fortified foods.
- Magnesium: Upholds muscle and nerve capability, energy creation, and bone wellbeing. Tracked down in nuts, seeds, entire grains, and mixed greens.
- Potassium: Regulates fluid balance, muscle contractions, and heart function. Found in bananas, potatoes, beans, and leafy greens.
- Sodium: Significant for liquid equilibrium, nerve capability, and muscle withdrawals. Tracked down in salt and many handled food sources.

Trace Minerals:

- Iron: Essential for oxygen transport in red blood cells and energy production. Found in meat, beans, fortified cereals, and leafy greens.
- Zinc: Upholds resistant capability, wound mending, and DNA union. Found in meat, shellfish, nuts, and whole grains.
- Selenium: Acts as an antioxidant, supporting thyroid function and immune health. Found in Brazil nuts, fish, and entire grains.
- Iodine: Necessary for thyroid hormone production and regulation. Found in iodized salt, seafood, and dairy products.

Importance in Carb Cycling

Nutrient Density: Consuming a variety of nutrient-dense foods ensures adequate intake of vitamins and minerals during carb cycling phases.

Metabolic Support: Micronutrients play crucial roles in energy metabolism, hormone regulation, and cellular function, supporting overall health and well-being.

Recovery and Performance: Vitamins and minerals aid in muscle recovery, immune function, and energy production, optimizing performance during high-intensity workouts and recovery periods.

Micronutrients, including vitamins and minerals, are essential for optimal health and performance during carb cycling. By emphasizing nutrient-dense foods rich in vitamins and minerals, individuals can support metabolic health, enhance energy levels, and promote overall well-being. Incorporating a variety of fruits, vegetables, lean proteins, and whole grains ensures a balanced intake of micronutrients, contributing to long-term health benefits and success in achieving fitness goals.

3.3 The Importance of Hydration

Hydration is a fundamental aspect of health and wellness, playing a crucial role in nearly every bodily function. Proper hydration is especially important when following a carb cycling diet, as it supports metabolic processes, exercise performance, and overall well-being.

Body Functions and Hydration

- Cellular Function: Water is essential for maintaining cellular homeostasis, facilitating biochemical reactions, and enabling nutrient transport and waste removal within cells.
- Temperature Regulation: Hydration helps regulate body temperature through sweating and respiration, which is vital during physical activity and in hot environments.
- Digestive Health: Adequate water intake aids digestion by helping to dissolve nutrients and move waste through the digestive tract, preventing constipation and promoting regular bowel movements.
- Joint and Muscle Function: Water acts as a lubricant and cushion for joints, muscles, and tissues, reducing the risk of injury and enhancing physical performance.

Hydration and Metabolism

- Metabolic Processes: Water is involved in metabolizing carbohydrates and fats into energy. Proper hydration supports metabolic functions, including the breakdown of nutrients and the production of energy.
- Appetite Regulation: Staying hydrated can help regulate appetite and reduce the likelihood of overeating, as thirst is sometimes mistaken for hunger.

Hydration During Carb Cycling

- Carbohydrate Storage: Carbohydrates are stored in the body as glycogen, which binds to water in the muscles and liver. High-carb days may increase water retention, while low-carb days might lead to a reduction in stored water. Proper hydration ensures that the body can efficiently manage these fluctuations.
- Electrolyte Balance: Electrolytes like sodium, potassium, and magnesium are crucial for maintaining fluid balance and preventing dehydration. Carb cycling, especially on low-carb days, can affect electrolyte levels, making it important to replenish these minerals through diet or supplementation.
- Exercise Performance: Hydration is critical for maintaining physical performance, as even mild dehydration can impair strength, endurance, and cognitive function. Ensuring adequate fluid intake before, during, and after workouts helps optimize performance and recovery.

Signs of Dehydration

- Mild Dehydration: Symptoms include dry mouth, thirst, decreased urine output, and dark-colored urine.
- Moderate Dehydration: Signs may include dry skin, headache, dizziness, and muscle cramps.
- Severe Dehydration: Severe dehydration can lead to confusion, rapid heartbeat, low blood pressure, and in extreme cases, organ failure.

Tips for Staying Hydrated

- Drink Regularly: Aim to drink water consistently throughout the day rather than waiting until you feel thirsty. Carry a water bottle to remind yourself to drink.
- Monitor Urine Color: Pale yellow urine typically indicates proper hydration, while dark yellow or amber suggests the need for more fluids.
- Hydrate Before, During, and After Exercise: Increase fluid intake before physical activity, and continue to drink water during and after exercise to replenish lost fluids.

- Incorporate Hydrating Foods: Foods with high water content, such as fruits (e.g., watermelon, oranges) and vegetables (e.g., cucumbers, lettuce), contribute to overall hydration.
- Limit Dehydrating Substances: Reduce the intake of diuretics such as caffeine and alcohol, as they can increase fluid loss.

Hydration is a key component of health, especially when following a carb cycling diet. Proper hydration supports metabolic processes, exercise performance, and overall well-being. By maintaining adequate fluid intake and paying attention to signs of dehydration, individuals can ensure their bodies function optimally, promoting better health and enhancing the benefits of their dietary and fitness efforts.

Chapter 4: Hormonal Changes and Metabolism

4.1 The Impact of Menopause on Metabolism

Menopause denotes a critical change in a lady's life, commonly happening between the ages of 45 and 55. During this period, the body undergoes various physiological changes, including a decline in reproductive hormones such as estrogen and progesterone. These hormonal shifts can have a profound impact on metabolism, body composition, and overall health.

Hormonal Changes and Metabolic Impact

1. Decline in Estrogen Levels:

Estrogen and Metabolism: Estrogen plays a vital role in regulating metabolism, insulin sensitivity, and fat distribution. A decline in estrogen levels can lead to metabolic slowdowns, making it more challenging to maintain a healthy weight.

Fat Distribution: Lower estrogen levels often result in a shift in fat storage from the hips and thighs to the abdominal area, increasing the risk of visceral fat accumulation. Visceral fat is associated with a higher risk of metabolic disorders, including insulin resistance and cardiovascular disease.

2. Decreased Muscle Mass:

Muscle Loss: With age and the onset of menopause, women tend to lose muscle mass (sarcopenia). Since muscle tissue is metabolically active, a reduction in muscle mass leads to a slower basal metabolic rate (BMR), meaning the body burns fewer calories at rest.

Impact on Weight: This decrease in muscle mass contributes to weight gain and difficulty in losing weight, even when maintaining the same dietary and exercise habits.

3. Changes in Insulin Sensitivity:

Insulin Resistance: Menopause can affect insulin sensitivity, leading to an increased risk of insulin resistance. Insulin resistance makes it harder for the body to use glucose effectively, which can result in elevated blood sugar levels and a higher likelihood of developing type 2 diabetes.

Blood Sugar Regulation: Fluctuations in blood sugar levels can lead to increased hunger and cravings, particularly for high-carbohydrate and sugary foods, complicating weight management efforts.

4. Alterations in Energy Expenditure:

Reduced Physical Activity: Many women experience a decrease in physical activity levels during and after menopause, either due to lifestyle changes or physical discomforts such as joint pain. Reduced activity further decreases overall energy expenditure.

Energy Balance: Maintaining energy balance (calories consumed versus calories expended) becomes more challenging, leading to potential weight gain and difficulties in weight loss.

Strategies to Mitigate Metabolic Changes

1. Strength Training:

Muscle Preservation: Incorporating regular strength training exercises helps preserve and build muscle mass, which can counteract the decline in metabolic rate. Strength training can include resistance exercises, weight lifting, or body-weight exercises.

Increased BMR: Maintaining or increasing muscle mass boosts basal metabolic rate, aiding in weight management and improving overall metabolic health.

2. Balanced Nutrition:

Nutrient-Dense Foods: Focus on consuming nutrient-dense foods that provide essential vitamins and minerals, such as fruits, vegetables, lean proteins, whole grains, and healthy fats.

Adequate Protein: Ensuring adequate protein intake supports muscle maintenance and repair, which is crucial for maintaining a healthy metabolism.

Moderate Carbohydrates: Carb cycling can help manage insulin sensitivity and support metabolic health. Balancing high-carb and low-carb days allows for flexibility in managing energy needs and hormonal fluctuations.

3. Regular Physical Activity:

Aerobic Exercise: Engage in regular aerobic exercises, such as walking, jogging, swimming, or cycling, to boost cardiovascular health and support calorie burning.

Flexibility and Balance: Incorporate flexibility and balance exercises, such as yoga or Pilates, to enhance overall physical function and reduce the risk of injuries.

4. Hormonal Balance:

Consult Healthcare Providers: Seek guidance from healthcare providers to manage hormonal imbalances. Hormone replacement therapy (HRT) or other medical interventions may be considered to alleviate menopausal symptoms and support metabolic health.

Stress Management: Implement stress-reducing techniques such as mindfulness, meditation, or deep breathing exercises to manage cortisol levels, which can affect metabolism and weight.

Menopause brings significant hormonal changes that can impact metabolism, leading to weight gain, changes in fat distribution, and increased risk of metabolic disorders. By understanding these changes and implementing strategies such as strength training, balanced nutrition, regular physical activity, and hormonal management, women can mitigate the adverse effects on metabolism and maintain overall health and well-being during and after menopause.

4.2 Hormonal Imbalances and Weight Gain

Hormonal imbalances during menopause can significantly affect a woman's metabolism and contribute to weight gain. The fluctuations in key hormones, such as estrogen, progesterone, and cortisol, play a critical role in regulating various bodily functions, including appetite, fat storage, and energy expenditure. Understanding these hormonal changes can help in managing weight effectively during this transitional phase of life.

Key Hormones and Their Roles
1. Estrogen:

Function: Estrogen helps regulate metabolism, insulin sensitivity, and fat distribution. It also plays a role in controlling appetite and energy balance.

Imbalance Effects: As estrogen levels decline during menopause, women may experience increased fat storage, particularly in the abdominal area. This shift in fat distribution is associated with a higher risk of metabolic syndrome and cardiovascular diseases.

2. Progesterone:

Function: Progesterone works alongside estrogen to maintain hormonal balance, support reproductive health, and regulate mood and sleep patterns.

Imbalance Effects: Decreasing progesterone levels can lead to water retention, bloating, and increased fat storage. Progesterone deficiency may also contribute to mood swings and sleep disturbances, indirectly affecting weight management by influencing stress and emotional eating.

3. Cortisol:

Function: Cortisol, known as the stress hormone, helps the body respond to stress and regulate metabolism, blood sugar levels, and immune function.

Imbalance Effects: Chronic stress and elevated cortisol levels can lead to increased appetite, cravings for high-calorie foods, and fat accumulation, particularly around the abdomen. High cortisol levels can also disrupt sleep patterns, further complicating weight management.

Insulin:

Function: Insulin is responsible for regulating blood sugar levels by facilitating the uptake of glucose into cells for energy or storage as fat.

Imbalance Effects: Insulin resistance, common during menopause, can result in elevated blood sugar levels and increased fat storage. This resistance can lead to type 2 diabetes if not managed properly.

Mechanisms of Hormonal Imbalance-Induced Weight Gain

1. Increased Appetite and Cravings:

- Hormonal imbalances can disrupt appetite-regulating hormones such as leptin and ghrelin, leading to increased hunger and cravings for sugary and high-fat foods. This can bring about gorging and ensuing weight gain.

2. Reduced Metabolic Rate:

- Lower levels of estrogen and progesterone can slow down the basal metabolic rate (BMR), reducing the number of calories burned at rest. A slower metabolism makes it easier to gain weight even with a consistent calorie intake.

3. Altered Fat Distribution:

- Hormonal changes during menopause often cause fat to be stored more readily in the abdominal region rather than the hips and thighs. This visceral fat is more metabolically active and associated with greater health risks compared to subcutaneous fat.

4. Impact on Sleep:

- Hormonal imbalances can disrupt sleep patterns, leading to poor quality or insufficient sleep. Sleep deprivation is linked to increased levels of ghrelin (hunger hormone) and decreased levels of leptin (satiety hormone), which can promote overeating and weight gain

Chapter 5: Getting Started with Carb Cycling

5.1 Assessing Your Current Diet and Lifestyle

Before embarking on a carb cycling regimen, it's essential to assess your current diet and lifestyle. Understanding your baseline habits will help you tailor a carb cycling plan that aligns with your goals, preferences, and nutritional needs. This assessment involves evaluating your dietary patterns, physical activity levels, and overall lifestyle choices to identify areas for improvement and set realistic goals.

Evaluating Your Dietary Habits

1. Food Diary:

- Purpose: Keeping a detailed food diary for a week can provide insights into your eating habits, portion sizes, and food choices.
- What to Track: Record everything you eat and drink, including meals, snacks, and beverages. Note the time of consumption, portion sizes, and any accompanying emotions or hunger levels.

2. Nutrient Intake:

- Macronutrients: Assess the balance of carbohydrates, proteins, and fats in your diet. Determine if you are consuming too many refined carbs or unhealthy fats and whether you're getting enough protein.
- Micronutrients: Evaluate your intake of essential vitamins and minerals. Ensure you are consuming a variety of fruits, vegetables, whole grains, and lean proteins to meet your micronutrient needs.

3. Eating Patterns:

- Meal Frequency: Note how often you eat throughout the day. Are you eating regular meals, or do you often skip meals and rely on snacks?
- Timing: Observe the timing of your meals and snacks. Are you eating late at night or going long periods without eating during the day?

4. Hydration:

- Fluid Intake: Track your daily water intake. Hold back nothing eight glasses of water each day, changing in light of your movement level and environment.
- Other Beverages: Note the consumption of other beverages like coffee, tea, sugary drinks, and alcohol. Excessive intake of these can impact your overall hydration and health.

Assessing Your Physical Activity

1. Exercise Frequency and Type:

- Current Routine: Document how often you exercise, the types of activities you engage in (e.g., cardio, strength training, flexibility exercises), and the duration of each session.
- Intensity: Assess the intensity of your workouts. Are you engaging in moderate to vigorous physical activity, or are your activities primarily low intensity?

2. Sedentary Behavior:

- Daily Movement: Note how much time you spend sitting or being inactive during the day. Prolonged sedentary behavior can negatively impact your metabolism and overall health.
- Breaks: Identify if you take regular breaks to stand up, stretch, or move around, especially if you have a desk job or spend a lot of time sitting.

Lifestyle Factors

1. Stress Levels:

- Sources of Stress: Identify common stressors in your life, such as work, family responsibilities, or financial concerns.
- Coping Mechanisms: Evaluate how you manage stress. Do you have healthy coping strategies, or do you rely on food, alcohol, or other unhealthy habits to cope?

2. Sleep Patterns:

- Sleep Duration: Assess the quantity and quality of your sleep. Go for the gold long stretches of rest each night to help by and large wellbeing and prosperity.
- Sleep Hygiene: Consider your sleep environment and habits. Are you maintaining a consistent sleep schedule, avoiding screens before bed, and creating a restful environment?

3. Social and Emotional Factors:

- Support System: Evaluate your social support network. Having supportive friends and family can positively influence your health and dietary choices.
- Emotional Eating: Distinguish on the off chance that you will more often than not eat in light of feelings like pressure, weariness, or misery. Emotional eating can hinder your ability to maintain a balanced diet.

Setting Goals and Making Adjustments

1. Identify Areas for Improvement:

- Dietary Changes: Based on your assessment, identify specific areas where you can improve your diet, such as reducing refined carbs, increasing protein intake, or adding more fruits and vegetables.

- Exercise Adjustments: Set realistic goals to increase your physical activity, whether by adding more exercise sessions, trying new activities, or increasing the intensity of your workouts.

2. Create an Action Plan:

- Specific Goals: Set specific, measurable, achievable, relevant, and time-bound (SMART) goals for your diet and lifestyle changes.
- Step-by-Step Plan: Develop a step-by-step plan to implement these changes gradually, allowing your body to adapt and making the process sustainable.

3. Monitor Progress:

- Track Changes: Continue to track your diet, exercise, and lifestyle habits to monitor your progress and make necessary adjustments.
- Celebrate Successes: Acknowledge and celebrate your achievements, no matter how small, to stay motivated and committed to your goals.

Assessing your current diet and lifestyle is a crucial first step in adopting a carb cycling plan. By understanding your baseline habits and identifying areas for improvement, you can create a personalized plan that supports your health and fitness goals. This comprehensive assessment will help you make informed decisions, set realistic goals, and achieve lasting changes for a healthier, more balanced life.

5.2 Setting Realistic Goals

Establishing achievable goals is crucial when adopting a carb cycling regimen, especially for women over 50. Realistic goals ensure that your expectations are practical and manageable, enhancing motivation and sustaining long-term commitment to your health journey. This section will guide you through the process of setting personalized, attainable goals that align with your lifestyle, preferences, and overall health objectives.

Understanding the Importance of Realistic Goals

1. Sustainability and Consistency:

Realistic goals promote sustainability, ensuring that changes to your diet and lifestyle are manageable over time.

Achievable goals foster consistency, allowing you to maintain positive habits without feeling overwhelmed or discouraged.

2. Motivation and Progress:

Attainable goals provide a sense of accomplishment as you achieve milestones, reinforcing motivation and encouraging continued progress.

Realistic expectations reduce pressure and allow you to celebrate incremental improvements along your health journey.

3. Flexibility and Adaptation:

Setting realistic goals allows for flexibility to adjust based on your body's responses, lifestyle changes, and unforeseen circumstances.

This adaptive approach ensures that your goals remain relevant and achievable as you navigate challenges and adjustments.

Steps to Setting Realistic Goals

1. Assess Your Starting Point:

- Evaluate your current diet, exercise routine, and lifestyle habits to understand where you are starting from.
- Consider factors like health status, physical activity levels, and dietary preferences to tailor goals that fit your unique circumstances.

2. Define Your Objectives:

- Clearly outline what you want to achieve with specific, measurable goals. Whether it's weight loss, improved energy levels, or better overall health, clarity helps you stay focused.
- Ensure your goals are measurable so that progress can be tracked and adjustments can be made as needed.

3. Break Goals into Manageable Steps:

- Set short-term goals that can be achieved within a few weeks to a couple of months. These smaller goals create stepping stones towards your larger objectives.
- Long-term goals should align with your overall vision for health and wellness, providing direction and motivation for sustained progress.

4. Ensure Goals Are Achievable:

- Consider your current lifestyle, commitments, and resources when setting goals to ensure they are realistic and within reach.
- Avoid setting goals that require drastic changes or unsustainable practices, as these can lead to frustration and setbacks.

5. Make Goals Relevant and Meaningful:

- Align your goals with your personal values, priorities, and motivations to increase their relevance and importance in your daily life.

- Connect your goals to tangible benefits, such as improved quality of life, enhanced well-being, or reduced health risks, to maintain motivation.

6. Set Time-Bound Goals:

- Assign specific timelines to your goals to create accountability and establish a sense of urgency for achievement.
- Break long-term goals into smaller milestones with clear deadlines to track progress and celebrate accomplishments along the way.

Practical Examples of Realistic Goals

1. Dietary Goals:

- Aim to include one additional serving of vegetables in your meals each day for the next month.
- Reduce consumption of sugary snacks by replacing them with healthier alternatives like fruits or nuts.

2. Exercise Goals:

- Commit to walking for 30 minutes, five times a week, for the next six weeks to increase physical activity.
- Incorporate two strength training sessions per week to build muscle and improve overall fitness.

3. Lifestyle Goals:

- Drink at least eight glasses of water daily for the next month to improve hydration and overall health.
- Establish a consistent sleep schedule by going to bed and waking up at the same time each day to enhance sleep quality.

4. Mental Health Goals:

- Practice mindfulness or meditation for 10 minutes daily to reduce stress and promote relaxation.
- Connect with a friend or family member at least once a week to foster social connections and support.

Monitoring and Adjusting Goals

1. Track Progress:

- Regularly review your goals and track progress using journals, apps, or progress charts to stay accountable and motivated.
- Celebrate achievements and milestones, no matter how small, to reinforce positive behaviors and maintain momentum.

2. Flexibility and Adaptation:

- Be open to adjusting your goals based on feedback from your body and changes in your circumstances or priorities.
- Modify goals that prove too challenging or unrealistic to ensure they remain achievable and supportive of your overall well-being.

Setting realistic goals is fundamental to the success of a carb cycling plan for women over 50. By assessing your current habits, defining specific and achievable objectives, and breaking them down into manageable steps, you can create a sustainable path to improved health and well-being. Remember to celebrate progress, stay flexible in your approach, and maintain a positive outlook as you work towards achieving your goals. With realistic goals in place, you are empowered to make lasting changes and enjoy a healthier, more fulfilling lifestyle.

5.3 Creating a Carb Cycling Plan

Creating a carb cycling plan tailored for women over 50 involves strategically alternating carbohydrate intake to optimize energy levels, metabolism, and overall health. This section will guide you through the process of designing a personalized carb cycling plan, taking into account your individual goals, preferences, and nutritional needs.

Understanding Carb Cycling

Carb cycling involves alternating between periods of higher and lower carbohydrate intake throughout the week. This approach is designed to optimize energy levels, support metabolic flexibility, and enhance fat loss while preserving muscle mass. For women over 50, carb cycling can be particularly beneficial in managing weight, hormone balance, and overall well-being.

Steps to Creating a Carb Cycling Plan

1. Assess Your Goals and Needs:

- Health Objectives: Determine your primary goals, whether it's weight management, improving energy levels, enhancing physical performance, or supporting overall health.
- Nutritional Needs: Consider any dietary preferences, food sensitivities, or medical conditions that may influence your carb cycling approach.

2. Determine Carb Cycling Patterns:

- Cycle Duration: Decide on the duration of each carb cycling cycle (e.g., daily, weekly). Common cycles include daily alternations or weekly cycles with high and low carb days.
- High Carb Days: Choose which days or meals will include higher carbohydrate intake to fuel intense workouts or higher energy demands.

- Low Carb Days: Plan days or meals with reduced carbohydrate intake to promote fat burning and improve insulin sensitivity.

3. Calculate Macronutrient Distribution:

- Carbohydrates: Determine the amount of carbohydrates you will consume on high and low carb days. High carb days may range from 1.5-2.5 grams of carbs per pound of body weight, while low carb days may be around 0.5 grams per pound.
- Proteins: Ensure adequate protein intake to support muscle maintenance and recovery, typically around 0.7-1 gram per pound of body weight.
- Fats: Include healthy fats to provide essential fatty acids and support overall health, making up the remaining calories after carbohydrates and proteins.

4. Plan Meals and Recipes:

- High Carb Day Meals: Create meal plans that include whole grains, fruits, and starchy vegetables to replenish glycogen stores and support energy-intensive activities.
- Low Carb Day Meals: Prepare meals with lean proteins, non-starchy vegetables, and healthy fats to promote satiety, stabilize blood sugar levels, and encourage fat burning.
- Snack Options: Include balanced snacks that align with your carb cycling goals, such as Greek yogurt with berries on high carb days or nuts and seeds on low carb days.

5. Hydration and Supplements:

- Hydration: Remain hydrated by drinking a lot of water over the course of the day. Consider adding electrolytes or sports drinks on high carb days, especially during intense workouts.

- Supplements: Consult with a healthcare provider to determine if supplements like vitamins, minerals, or protein powders are necessary to support your carb cycling plan and overall health.

6. Monitor Progress and Adjustments:

- Track Results: Keep a journal or use a tracking app to monitor how your body responds to carb cycling. Note changes in energy levels, mood, performance, and body composition.
- Adjust as Needed: Be flexible and adjust your carb cycling plan based on feedback from your body and progress towards your goals. Modify carbohydrate intake, meal timing, or cycle duration as necessary.

Sample Carb Cycling Plan Outline

1. Weekly Schedule:

Day 1 (High Carb): Include higher carbohydrate foods like whole grains, fruits, and legumes.

Day 2 (Low Carb): Focus on lean proteins, leafy greens, and healthy fats with minimal carbohydrates.

Day 3 (Moderate Carb): Balance carbohydrates, proteins, and fats to support moderate activity levels.

Repeat Cycle: Continue alternating high, low, and moderate carb days throughout the week.

2. Meal Examples:

Breakfast (High Carb): Oatmeal with berries and a side of Greek yogurt.

Lunch (Low Carb): Grilled chicken salad with mixed greens, avocado, and olive oil dressing.

Dinner (Moderate Carb): Baked salmon with quinoa and roasted vegetables.

3. Snack Options:

High Carb Day: Banana with almond butter, whole grain toast with avocado.
Low Carb Day: Cottage cheese with cucumber slices, hard-boiled eggs.

Designing a carb cycling plan for women over 50 requires careful consideration of individual goals, preferences, and nutritional needs. By strategically alternating carbohydrate intake based on high, low, and moderate carb days, you can optimize energy levels, support metabolic health, and achieve your health and fitness objectives. Remember to monitor your progress, stay flexible in your approach, and seek guidance from healthcare professionals as needed to ensure your carb cycling plan aligns with your overall well-being.

5.4 Tracking Your Progress

Tracking your progress is essential when adopting a carb cycling regimen for women over 50. Monitoring your journey allows you to assess the effectiveness of your approach, stay motivated, and make informed adjustments to achieve your health and fitness goals. This section outlines practical strategies for tracking progress and staying on course with your carb cycling plan.

Importance of Tracking Progress

1. Accountability and Motivation:

- Tracking your progress creates accountability, helping you stay committed to your health goals and maintain consistency in your carb cycling plan.
- Seeing tangible results over time provides motivation to continue making healthy choices and pushing towards your desired outcomes.

2. Identifying What Works:

- Monitoring your progress allows you to identify which aspects of your carb cycling plan are effective in achieving your goals, such as improved energy levels, weight management, or enhanced physical performance.
- It enables you to make data-driven decisions about adjustments to your diet, exercise routine, or overall lifestyle.

3. Adjusting Your Approach:

- Tracking allows you to recognize patterns and trends in your progress, such as fluctuations in energy levels or changes in body composition, prompting you to adjust your carb cycling plan accordingly.
- It provides insights into how your body responds to different macronutrient ratios, meal timings, and exercise intensity levels, optimizing your overall health and well-being.

Strategies for Tracking Progress

1. Keep a Food Journal:

- Record daily food intake, including the types and quantities of carbohydrates, proteins, fats, and calories consumed.
- Note meal timings, portion sizes, and any snacks or beverages to maintain awareness of your dietary habits.

2. Track Physical Activity:

- Monitor your exercise sessions, including duration, intensity, and types of activities performed.
- Keep a log of workouts, steps taken, or other physical activities to gauge your overall activity level and calorie expenditure.

3. Measure Body Metrics:

- Regularly measure key body metrics such as weight, body fat percentage, waist circumference, and muscle mass.
- Track changes in these metrics over time to assess progress towards your health and fitness goals.

4. Use Technology and Apps:

- Utilize mobile apps or online tools designed for tracking nutrition, exercise, and health metrics.
- These tools can provide visual graphs, charts, and summaries of your progress, making it easier to monitor trends and make informed decisions.

5. Assess Energy Levels and Well-Being:

- Pay attention to changes in energy levels, mood, sleep quality, and overall well-being throughout your carb cycling journey.

- Note any improvements or challenges related to your dietary choices, exercise routine, or lifestyle habits.

6. Regular Self-Assessment:

- Schedule periodic self-assessments to reflect on your progress, achievements, and areas for improvement.
- Celebrate milestones and accomplishments to maintain motivation and reinforce positive behaviors.

Adjusting Your Carb Cycling Plan

1. Evaluate Progress Regularly:

- Review your tracking data regularly to assess your progress towards achieving your health and fitness goals.
- Identify strengths and areas for improvement in your carb cycling plan based on the insights gained from tracking.

2. Make Informed Adjustments:

- Use your tracking data to make informed adjustments to your carb cycling plan, such as modifying macronutrient ratios, adjusting meal timing, or refining exercise routines.
- Consult with healthcare professionals or nutrition experts as needed to ensure adjustments align with your health objectives.

3. Set New Goals:

- Based on your progress and insights, set new goals to continue challenging yourself and advancing towards improved health and well-being.
- Establish realistic and achievable goals that build upon your current achievements and maintain momentum in your carb cycling journey.

Tracking your progress is a valuable tool for maximizing the benefits of carb cycling and achieving your health goals as a woman over 50. By maintaining accountability, identifying effective strategies, and making informed adjustments, you can optimize your dietary choices, physical activity, and overall well-being. Embrace tracking as a supportive tool on your journey towards sustainable health and enjoy the rewards of a balanced and fulfilling lifestyle.

Chapter 6: Carb Cycling Meal Plans

6.1 High-Carb Days: What to Eat

High-carb days are a crucial component of the carb cycling plan, designed to replenish glycogen stores, support muscle recovery, and provide energy for intense physical activities. For women over 50, high-carb days can also help balance hormones and improve overall well-being. This section will guide you on what to eat on high-carb days to maximize the benefits of carb cycling.

The Role of High-Carb Days

1. Replenishing Glycogen Stores:

- High-carb days replenish glycogen stores in the muscles and liver, providing the necessary energy for physical activities and preventing fatigue.
- Glycogen is the primary fuel source for high-intensity and endurance exercises, making high-carb days essential for active individuals.

2. Supporting Hormonal Balance:

- Carbohydrates play a role in regulating hormones, including insulin and cortisol, which are crucial for maintaining energy levels and overall health.
- For women over 50, balanced hormone levels can improve mood, reduce stress, and support metabolic health.

3. Enhancing Muscle Recovery and Growth:

- Adequate carbohydrate intake on high-carb days supports muscle recovery and growth by providing the necessary energy and nutrients for repair and regeneration.

- High-carb days can help prevent muscle breakdown and promote lean muscle mass, which is important for maintaining strength and metabolic rate.

What to Eat on High-Carb Days

1. Whole Grains:

- Oats: An incredible wellspring of mind boggling carbs, fiber, and fundamental supplements. Enjoy oatmeal topped with fruits and nuts for a nutritious breakfast.
- Brown Rice: Provides sustained energy and pairs well with lean proteins and vegetables for a balanced meal.
- Quinoa: A complete protein source that is also rich in carbohydrates and fiber, perfect for salads, bowls, and side dishes.

2. Fruits:

- Berries: Rich in antioxidants, vitamins, and fiber. Add them to yogurt, smoothies, or mixed greens for an invigorating and nutritious lift.
- Bananas: High in potassium and carbohydrates, ideal for a quick energy boost before or after workouts.
- Apples and Oranges: Provide vitamins, fiber, and natural sugars to keep you energized throughout the day.

3. Starchy Vegetables:

- Sweet Potatoes: Packed with vitamins, minerals, and fiber. Roast or bake them as a side dish or add them to salads and bowls.
- Squash: Versatile and nutrient-dense, great for soups, stews, or as a roasted vegetable side.
- Corn: Provides carbohydrates and fiber. Enjoy it as part of salads, soups, or as a grilled side dish.

4. Legumes:

- Lentils: High in protein, fiber, and complex carbohydrates. Use them in soups, stews, or salads for a filling and nutritious meal.
- Chickpeas: Versatile and nutrient-rich, perfect for hummus, salads, or roasted as a snack.
- Black Beans: Provide protein, fiber, and carbohydrates. Add them to rice dishes, tacos, or salads for a balanced meal.

5. Dairy and Dairy Alternatives:

- Greek Yogurt: High in protein and carbohydrates. Top with fruits, nuts, and honey for a delicious and satisfying snack or breakfast.
- Milk and Plant-Based Milks: Provide carbohydrates, protein, and essential nutrients. Use them in smoothies, cereals, or as a beverage.

6. Healthy Snacks:

- Whole Grain Crackers: Pair with hummus, guacamole, or cheese for a balanced snack.
- Energy Bars: Choose bars made with whole grains, nuts, and natural sweeteners for a convenient and nutritious option.
- Rice Cakes: Top with nut butter, avocado, or cottage cheese for a light and energizing snack.

Meal Planning Tips for High-Carb Days

Balance Macronutrients:

- Ensure your meals include a balance of carbohydrates, proteins, and fats to provide sustained energy and support overall health.

- Combine high-carb foods with lean proteins and healthy fats to create satisfying and nutritious meals.

Portion Control:

- Be aware of part sizes to keep away from overconsumption of calories. Aim to fill half your plate with high-carb foods, a quarter with lean proteins, and the remaining quarter with vegetables and healthy fats.

Meal Timing:

- Distribute your carbohydrate intake evenly throughout the day to maintain steady energy levels and prevent blood sugar spikes.
- Consider consuming higher-carb meals around your workouts to fuel performance and aid in recovery.

Hydration:

- Stay hydrated by drinking plenty of water throughout the day. Legitimate hydration upholds processing, digestion, and generally prosperity.

High-carb days are an integral part of carb cycling, providing the energy and nutrients needed for optimal performance, muscle recovery, and hormonal balance. By incorporating a variety of whole grains, fruits, starchy vegetables, legumes, dairy, and healthy snacks into your high-carb days, you can enjoy nutritious and satisfying meals that support your health goals. Plan your meals thoughtfully, balance your macronutrients, and stay hydrated to make the most of your high-carb days and enhance your overall well-being.

6.2 Low-Carb Days: What to Eat

Low-carb days are an essential component of the carb cycling plan, particularly beneficial for promoting fat loss, enhancing insulin sensitivity, and supporting overall metabolic health. For women over 50, low-carb days can help manage weight, stabilize blood sugar levels, and improve energy balance. This section will guide you on what to eat on low-carb days to optimize these benefits.

The Role of Low-Carb Days

1. Promoting Fat Loss:

- Reducing carbohydrate intake encourages the body to utilize stored fat for energy, aiding in fat loss and weight management.
- Low-carb days help deplete glycogen stores, prompting the body to burn fat more efficiently.

2. Enhancing Insulin Sensitivity:

- Lowering carbohydrate consumption can improve insulin sensitivity, helping to regulate blood sugar levels and reduce the risk of insulin resistance.
- Stable blood sugar levels contribute to better energy balance and reduced cravings.

3. Supporting Metabolic Health:

- Low-carb diets have been associated with improved lipid profiles, including lower triglycerides and higher HDL cholesterol.
- For women over 50, these benefits can contribute to better heart health and overall metabolic well-being.

What to Eat on Low-Carb Days

1. Lean Proteins:

- Chicken Breast: A lean source of protein, perfect for salads, stir-fries, and grilled dishes.
- Turkey: Versatile and low in fat, ideal for a variety of recipes from sandwiches to roasted meals.
- Fish: High in protein and healthy fats, options like salmon, cod, and tilapia are excellent for low-carb meals.
- Eggs: Rich in protein and essential nutrients, eggs can be enjoyed boiled, scrambled, or in omelets.

2. Non-Starchy Vegetables:

- Leafy Greens: Spinach, kale, and arugula are low in carbs and high in vitamins, minerals, and fiber. Use them in salads, smoothies, and sautés.
- Cruciferous Vegetables: Broccoli, cauliflower, and Brussels sprouts are nutrient-dense and low in carbohydrates, perfect for roasting or steaming.
- Peppers and Zucchini: Versatile and low in carbs, great for grilling, stir-fries, or adding to salads.
- Mushrooms: Low in carbs and calories, mushrooms add flavor and texture to various dishes.

3. Healthy Fats:

- Avocado: High in healthy monounsaturated fats, avocados can be added to salads, smoothies, or enjoyed as a spread.
- Nuts and Seeds: Almonds, walnuts, chia seeds, and flaxseeds provide healthy fats, protein, and fiber. Use them as snacks or toppings for yogurt and salads.
- Olive Oil: Rich in monounsaturated fats, olive oil is ideal for dressings, cooking, and drizzling over vegetables.
- Coconut Oil: A source of medium-chain triglycerides (MCTs), coconut oil can be used for cooking or adding to smoothies and coffee.

4. Dairy and Dairy Alternatives:

- Greek Yogurt: Low in carbs and high in protein. Choose plain, unsweetened varieties and add low-carb toppings like berries or nuts.
- Cheese: Cheese varieties such as cheddar, mozzarella, and feta are low in carbs and can be added to salads, omelets, or eaten as snacks.
- Unsweetened Almond Milk: A low-carb alternative to regular milk, suitable for smoothies, coffee, and recipes.

5. Low-Carb Snacks:

- Vegetable Sticks with Dip: Carrot sticks, cucumber slices, and bell pepper strips paired with hummus, guacamole, or Greek yogurt dip.
- Hard-Boiled Eggs: A convenient and protein-rich snack that's easy to prepare and carry.
- Cheese and Nut Mix: A combination of cheese cubes and a handful of nuts for a balanced, low-carb snack.
- Seaweed Snacks: Low in carbs and calories, seaweed snacks provide a crunchy and nutritious option.

Meal Planning Tips for Low-Carb Days

1. Balance Macronutrients:

- Focus on high-quality proteins and healthy fats to keep you full and satisfied throughout the day.
- Incorporate plenty of non-starchy vegetables to add volume and nutrients to your meals without excess carbs.

2. Portion Control:

- Be mindful of portion sizes, especially with calorie-dense foods like nuts and seeds, to avoid overconsumption.

- Aim to fill half your plate with vegetables, a quarter with lean proteins, and the remaining quarter with healthy fats.

3. Meal Timing:

- Distribute your meals and snacks evenly throughout the day to maintain steady energy levels and prevent hunger.
- Consider having a protein-rich snack or meal before and after workouts to support muscle recovery and energy balance.

4. Hydration:

- Drink a lot of water over the course of the day to remain hydrated and support processing and digestion.
- Natural teas and implanted water can mix it up and flavor to your hydration schedule.

Low-carb days are a vital part of carb cycling, promoting fat loss, enhancing insulin sensitivity, and supporting overall metabolic health. By incorporating a variety of lean proteins, non-starchy vegetables, healthy fats, and low-carb snacks, you can enjoy nutritious and satisfying meals that align with your health goals. Plan your meals carefully, balance your macronutrients, and stay hydrated to make the most of your low-carb days and optimize your well-being.

6.3 Sample Weekly Meal Plan

Day 1: High-Carb Day

Breakfast:

- Greek yogurt parfait with mixed berries, honey, and granola.

Snack:

- Apple slices with almond butter.

Lunch:

- Quinoa salad with chickpeas, cherry tomatoes, cucumbers, feta cheese, and a lemon-tahini dressing.

Snack:

- Rice cakes topped with avocado and cherry tomatoes.

Dinner:

- Grilled chicken breast with brown rice, steamed broccoli, and a side of roasted sweet potatoes.

Day 2: Low-Carb Day

Breakfast:

- Scrambled eggs with spinach, mushrooms, and feta cheese.

Snack:

- Celery sticks with hummus.

Lunch:

- Grilled salmon salad with mixed greens, cucumbers, bell peppers, and a vinaigrette dressing.

Snack:

- Hard-boiled eggs.

Dinner:

- Beef stir-fry with broccoli, bell peppers, and snow peas, served over cauliflower rice.

Day 3: High-Carb Day

Breakfast:

- Oatmeal topped with sliced bananas, walnuts, and a drizzle of maple syrup.

Snack:

- Pear slices with cottage cheese.

Lunch:

- Whole grain wrap with turkey, avocado, lettuce, and tomato.

Snack:

- Carrot sticks with guacamole.

Dinner:

- Baked cod with quinoa, roasted Brussels sprouts, and a side of butternut squash.

Day 4: Low-Carb Day

Breakfast:

- Smoothie with unsweetened almond milk, spinach, avocado, protein powder, and chia seeds.

Snack:

- Cheese cubes and a handful of almonds.

Lunch:

- Chicken Caesar salad with romaine lettuce, grilled chicken, Parmesan cheese, and Caesar dressing.

Snack:

- Greek yogurt with a few raspberries.

Dinner:

- Pork tenderloin with sautéed green beans and a side of mashed cauliflower.

Day 5: High-Carb Day

Breakfast:

- Whole grain toast with almond butter and sliced strawberries.

Snack:

- Orange slices and a small handful of walnuts.

Lunch:

- Brown rice bowl with black beans, corn, tomatoes, avocado, and cilantro lime dressing.

Snack:

- Greek yogurt with granola and blueberries.

Dinner:

- Shrimp stir-fry with mixed vegetables and jasmine rice.

Day 6: Low-Carb Day

Breakfast:

- Omelet with tomatoes, bell peppers, onions, and cheese.

Snack:

- Sliced cucumbers with tzatziki.

Lunch:

- Turkey lettuce wraps with avocado, shredded carrots, and a dollop of salsa.

Snack:

- Mixed nuts.

Dinner:

- Baked chicken thighs with roasted asparagus and a side of zucchini noodles.

Day 7: High-Carb Day

Breakfast:

- Smoothie bowl with mixed fruits, granola, and chia seeds.

Snack:

- Apple with a small handful of cashews.

Lunch:

- Lentil soup with whole grain bread.

Snack:

- Rice cakes with peanut butter and banana slices.

Dinner:

- Grilled tofu with brown rice, steamed green beans, and a side of roasted carrots.

6.4 Grocery Shopping Guide

Essentials for High-Carb Days

Whole Grains:

- Oats
- Brown rice
- Quinoa
- Whole grain bread
- Whole grain pasta

Fruits:

- Berries (strawberries, blueberries, raspberries)
- Bananas
- Apples
- Oranges
- Pears

Starchy Vegetables:

- Sweet potatoes
- Squash (butternut, acorn)
- Corn
- Peas

Legumes:

- Lentils
- Chickpeas
- Black beans
- Kidney beans

Dairy and Dairy Alternatives:

- Greek yogurt
- Milk (or plant-based alternatives like almond milk, soy milk)
- Cottage cheese

Healthy Snacks:

- Rice cakes
- Whole grain crackers
- Energy bars made with whole grains and nuts

Essentials for Low-Carb Days

Lean Proteins:

- Chicken breast
- Turkey breast
- Fish (salmon, cod, tilapia)
- Eggs
- Lean cuts of beef (sirloin, tenderloin)

Non-Starchy Vegetables:

- Leafy greens (spinach, kale, arugula)
- Cruciferous vegetables (broccoli, cauliflower, Brussels sprouts)
- Bell peppers
- Zucchini
- Mushrooms

Healthy Fats:

- Avocados
- Nuts (almonds, walnuts)
- Seeds (chia seeds, flaxseeds)
- Olive oil
- Coconut oil

Dairy and Dairy Alternatives:

- Cheese (cheddar, mozzarella, feta)
- Unsweetened Greek yogurt
- Unsweetened almond milk

Low-Carb Snacks:

- Vegetable sticks (carrots, celery, cucumber) with hummus
- Hard-boiled eggs
- Cheese cubes
- Seaweed snacks
- Pantry Staples

Condiments and Spices:

- Olive oil
- Coconut oil
- Vinegar (balsamic, apple cider)
- Soy sauce or tamari
- Mustard
- Herbs and spices (basil, oregano, cumin, paprika)

Nuts and Seeds:

- Almonds

- Walnuts
- Chia seeds
- Flaxseeds

Canned Goods:

- Canned tomatoes
- Canned beans (black beans, chickpeas)
- Canned tuna or salmon

Beverages:

- Herbal teas
- Green tea
- Coffee
- Sparkling water
- Fresh Produce

Vegetables:

- Leafy greens (spinach, kale, arugula)
- Cruciferous vegetables (broccoli, cauliflower, Brussels sprouts)
- Root vegetables (carrots, beets)
- Allium vegetables (onions, garlic)
- Peppers (bell peppers, chili peppers)
- Tomatoes
- Cucumbers
- Zucchini

Fruits:

- Berries (strawberries, blueberries, raspberries)
- Citrus fruits (oranges, lemons, limes)
- Apples

- Pears
- Bananas (for high-carb days)

Frozen Foods

Vegetables:

- Frozen broccoli
- Frozen spinach
- Frozen mixed vegetables

Fruits:

- Frozen berries
- Frozen mango
- Frozen pineapple

Proteins:

- Frozen chicken breast
- Frozen fish fillets
- Frozen shrimp

Chapter 7: Recipes

7.1 Breakfast Ideas

High-Carb Breakfast Ideas

1. Greek Yogurt Parfait
Ingredients:

- 1 cup Greek yogurt
- 1/2 cup mixed berries (strawberries, blueberries, raspberries)
- 1/4 cup granola
- 1 tablespoon honey

Directions:

1. Layer Greek yogurt, mixed berries, and granola in a bowl or glass.
2. Drizzle honey on top.
3. Serve immediately.

Serving:

1 serving
Nutrition:

Calories: 300
Carbohydrates: 45g
Protein: 15g
Fat: 8g

2. Oatmeal with Banana and Walnuts

Ingredients:

- 1 cup rolled oats
- 2 cups water or milk
- 1 banana, sliced
- 2 tablespoons walnuts, chopped
- 1 tablespoon maple syrup

Directions:

- Cook oats in water or milk according to package instructions.
- Top with banana slices, walnuts, and maple syrup.
- Serve warm.

Serving:

2 servings

Nutrition (per serving):

Calories: 350
Carbohydrates: 55g
Protein: 8g
Fat: 12g

3. Whole Grain Toast with Almond Butter and Strawberries

Ingredients:

- 2 slices whole grain bread
- 2 tablespoons almond butter
- 1/2 cup strawberries, sliced

Directions:

- Toast the bread.
- Spread almond butter on each slice.
- Top with sliced strawberries.
- Serve immediately.

Serving:

1 serving

Nutrition:

Calories: 350

Carbohydrates: 40g

Protein: 12g

Fat: 16g

4. Quinoa Breakfast Bowl

Ingredients:

- 1 cup cooked quinoa
- 1/2 cup almond milk
- 1 tablespoon chia seeds
- 1/2 cup blueberries
- 1 tablespoon honey

Directions:

1. Combine quinoa, almond milk, and chia seeds in a bowl.
2. Top with blueberries and drizzle honey.
3. Serve chilled or warm.

Serving:

2 servings
Nutrition (per serving):

Calories: 300
Carbohydrates: 50g
Protein: 8g
Fat: 8g

5. Smoothie Bowl
Ingredients:

- 1 banana, frozen
- 1/2 cup frozen mixed berries
- 1/2 cup Greek yogurt
- 1/2 cup almond milk
- 1 tablespoon chia seeds
- 1/4 cup granola

Directions:

1. Blend banana, mixed berries, Greek yogurt, and almond milk until smooth.
2. Pour into a bowl and top with chia seeds and granola.
3. Serve immediately.

Serving:

1 serving
Nutrition:

Calories: 400

Carbohydrates: 60g

Protein: 15g

Fat: 12g

6. Peanut Butter Banana Smoothie

Ingredients:

- 1 banana
- 1 tablespoon peanut butter
- 1 cup almond milk
- 1 tablespoon chia seeds
- 1 teaspoon honey

Directions:

1. Blend all ingredients until smooth.
2. Serve immediately.

Serving:

1 serving

Nutrition:

Calories: 350

Carbohydrates: 50g

Protein: 10g

Fat: 12g

7. Apple Cinnamon Overnight Oats

Ingredients:

- 1 cup rolled oats

- 1 cup almond milk
- 1 apple, chopped
- 1 teaspoon cinnamon
- 1 tablespoon maple syrup

Directions:

1. Combine oats, almond milk, apple, cinnamon, and maple syrup in a jar.
2. Refrigerate overnight.
3. Serve chilled.

Serving:

2 servings

Nutrition (per serving):

Calories: 300

Carbohydrates: 55g

Protein: 6g

Fat: 6g

Low-Carb Breakfast Ideas

1. Scrambled Eggs with Spinach and Mushrooms

Ingredients:

- 3 eggs
- 1 cup spinach, chopped
- 1/2 cup mushrooms, sliced
- 1 tablespoon olive oil
- Salt and pepper to taste

Directions:

1. Heat olive oil in a pan over medium heat.
2. Add mushrooms and cook until soft.
3. Add spinach and cook until wilted.
4. Whisk eggs, pour into the pan, and scramble until fully cooked.
5. Season with salt and pepper.

Serving:

1 serving

Nutrition:

Calories: 250

Carbohydrates: 5g

Protein: 18g

Fat: 18g

2. Avocado and Bacon Omelet

Ingredients:

- 3 eggs
- 1/2 avocado, sliced
- 2 slices bacon, cooked and crumbled
- 1 tablespoon butter
- Salt and pepper to taste

Directions:

1. Whisk eggs in a bowl.
2. Heat butter in a pan over medium heat.

3. Pour eggs into the pan and cook until set.

4. Add avocado and bacon on one half of the omelet.

5. Fold the omelet and serve.

Serving:

1 serving

Nutrition:

Calories: 350

Carbohydrates: 5g

Protein: 18g

Fat: 30g

3. Greek Yogurt with Nuts and Seeds

Ingredients:

- 1 cup Greek yogurt
- 2 tablespoons mixed nuts (almonds, walnuts)
- 1 tablespoon chia seeds
- 1 tablespoon flaxseeds
- 1 teaspoon honey

Directions:

1. Combine Greek yogurt, nuts, chia seeds, and flaxseeds in a bowl.

2. Drizzle honey on top.

3. Serve immediately.

Serving:

1 serving

Nutrition:

Calories: 300
Carbohydrates: 10g
Protein: 20g
Fat: 20g

4. Cottage Cheese and Cucumber Slices

Ingredients:

- 1 cup cottage cheese
- 1/2 cucumber, sliced
- Salt and pepper to taste

Directions:

1. Serve cottage cheese with cucumber slices on the side.
2. Season with salt and pepper.

Serving:

1 serving

Nutrition:

Calories: 200
Carbohydrates: 10g
Protein: 20g
Fat: 10g

5. Smoked Salmon and Avocado Plate

Ingredients:

- 2 ounces smoked salmon
- 1/2 avocado, sliced
- 1 cup mixed greens
- 1 tablespoon olive oil
- 1 teaspoon lemon juice
- Salt and pepper to taste

Directions:

1. Arrange smoked salmon, avocado, and mixed greens on a plate.
2. Drizzle with olive oil and lemon juice.
3. Season with salt and pepper.

Serving:

1 serving

Nutrition:

Calories: 250
Carbohydrates: 5g
Protein: 15g
Fat: 20g

6. Chia Seed Pudding

Ingredients:

- 1/4 cup chia seeds
- 1 cup unsweetened almond milk

- 1 teaspoon vanilla extract
- 1 tablespoon almond butter
- Berries for topping

Directions:

1. Combine chia seeds, almond milk, and vanilla extract in a bowl.
2. Refrigerate overnight.
3. Top with almond butter and berries before serving.

Serving:

2 servings

Nutrition (per serving):

Calories: 200

Carbohydrates: 10g

Protein: 6g

Fat: 15g

7. Egg Muffins with Vegetables

Ingredients:

- 6 eggs
- 1/2 cup bell peppers, diced
- 1/2 cup spinach, chopped
- 1/4 cup cheese, shredded
- Salt and pepper to taste

Directions:

1. Preheat oven to 375°F (190°C).
2. Whisk eggs in a bowl and add bell peppers, spinach, cheese, salt, and pepper.

3. Pour the mixture into a greased muffin tin.

4. Bake for 20 minutes or until eggs are set.

Serving:

6 muffins

Nutrition (per muffin):

Calories: 100

Carbohydrates: 2g

Protein: 8g

Fat: 7g

7.2 Lunch Recipes

High-Carb Lunch Recipes

1. Quinoa Salad with Chickpeas and Vegetables

Ingredients:

- 1 cup cooked quinoa
- 1 cup chickpeas, drained and rinsed
- 1 cup cherry tomatoes, halved
- 1 cucumber, diced
- 1/4 cup red onion, diced
- 1/4 cup feta cheese, crumbled
- 2 tablespoons olive oil
- 1 tablespoon lemon juice
- Salt and pepper to taste

Directions:

1. In a large bowl, combine quinoa, chickpeas, cherry tomatoes, cucumber, red onion, and feta cheese.
2. Drizzle with olive oil and lemon juice.
3. Toss to combine and season with salt and pepper.
4. Serve chilled.

Serving:

2 servings

Nutrition (per serving):

Calories: 350

Carbohydrates: 50g

Protein: 12g

Fat: 12g

2. Sweet Potato and Black Bean Burrito

Ingredients:

- 1 large sweet potato, peeled and diced
- 1 cup black beans, drained and rinsed
- 1/2 cup corn kernels
- 1/4 cup red onion, diced
- 1/2 cup salsa
- 1/2 cup shredded cheese
- 2 whole wheat tortillas

Directions:

1. Cook sweet potato in a skillet over medium heat until tender.
2. Add black beans, corn, and red onion to the skillet and cook until heated through.
3. Divide the mixture between the tortillas.
4. Top with salsa and shredded cheese.
5. Roll up the tortillas and serve.

Serving:

2 servings

Nutrition (per serving):

Calories: 400

Carbohydrates: 65g

Protein: 15g

Fat: 12g

3. Whole Grain Pasta with Marinara and Veggies

Ingredients:

- 2 cups cooked whole grain pasta
- 1 cup marinara sauce
- 1 zucchini, sliced
- 1 bell pepper, diced
- 1/4 cup grated Parmesan cheese
- 1 tablespoon olive oil
- Salt and pepper to taste

Directions:

1. Heat olive oil in a skillet over medium heat.
2. Add zucchini and bell pepper and cook until tender.
3. Add marinara sauce and cook until heated through.
4. Toss the sauce with the cooked pasta.
5. Sprinkle with Parmesan cheese and serve.

Serving:

2 servings

Nutrition (per serving):

Calories: 350

Carbohydrates: 55g

Protein: 12g

Fat: 10g

4. Lentil and Vegetable Stew

Ingredients:

- 1 cup lentils, rinsed
- 1 carrot, diced
- 1 celery stalk, diced
- 1 onion, diced
- 2 cups vegetable broth
- 1 cup diced tomatoes
- 1 teaspoon cumin
- 1 teaspoon paprika
- Salt and pepper to taste

Directions:

1. In a large pot, combine lentils, carrot, celery, onion, and vegetable broth.
2. Bring to a boil, then reduce heat and simmer until lentils are tender.
3. Add diced tomatoes, cumin, paprika, salt, and pepper.
4. Simmer for another 10 minutes and serve.

Serving:

2 servings

Nutrition (per serving):

Calories: 300

Carbohydrates: 50g

Protein: 15g

Fat: 2g

5. Brown Rice and Vegetable Stir-Fry

Ingredients:

- 2 cups cooked brown rice
- 1 cup broccoli florets
- 1 bell pepper, sliced
- 1 carrot, sliced
- 2 tablespoons soy sauce
- 1 tablespoon sesame oil
- 1 garlic clove, minced

Directions:

1. Heat sesame oil in a skillet over medium heat.
2. Add garlic and cook until fragrant.
3. Add broccoli, bell pepper, and carrot and cook until tender.
4. Add cooked brown rice and soy sauce.
5. Toss to combine and serve.

Serving:

2 servings

Nutrition (per serving):

Calories: 350

Carbohydrates: 60g

Protein: 8g

Fat: 10g

6. Chicken and Sweet Potato Bowl

Ingredients:

- 1 cup cooked quinoa
- 1 cup roasted sweet potato cubes
- 1 cup cooked chicken breast, diced
- 1/2 avocado, sliced
- 2 tablespoons olive oil
- 1 tablespoon lemon juice
- Salt and pepper to taste

Directions:

1. Combine quinoa, sweet potato, and chicken in a bowl.
2. Top with avocado slices.
3. Drizzle with olive oil and lemon juice.
4. Season with salt and pepper and serve.

Serving:

2 servings

Nutrition (per serving):

Calories: 400

Carbohydrates: 45g

Protein: 25g

Fat: 15g

7. Hummus and Veggie Wrap

Ingredients:

- 1 whole wheat tortilla

- 1/2 cup hummus
- 1/2 cup sliced cucumber
- 1/2 cup shredded carrot
- 1/4 cup spinach leaves
- 1/4 cup bell pepper, sliced

Directions:

1. Spread hummus evenly over the tortilla.
2. Layer cucumber, carrot, spinach, and bell pepper on top.
3. Roll up the tortilla and slice in half.
4. Serve immediately.

Serving:

1 serving

Nutrition:

Calories: 350
Carbohydrates: 50g
Protein: 10g
Fat: 12g

Low-Carb Lunch Recipes

1. Grilled Chicken Salad
Ingredients:

- 1 cup mixed greens
- 1/2 cup cherry tomatoes, halved
- 1/4 cup cucumber, sliced
- 1/4 cup red onion, sliced

- 1 grilled chicken breast, sliced
- 2 tablespoons olive oil
- 1 tablespoon balsamic vinegar
- Salt and pepper to taste

Directions:

1. In a large bowl, combine mixed greens, cherry tomatoes, cucumber, and red onion.
2. Top with grilled chicken slices.
3. Drizzle with olive oil and balsamic vinegar.
4. Toss to combine and season with salt and pepper.
5. Serve immediately.

Serving:

1 serving

Nutrition:

Calories: 300

Carbohydrates: 10g

Protein: 30g

Fat: 15g

2. Zucchini Noodles with Pesto

Ingredients:

- 2 medium zucchinis, spiralized
- 1/4 cup pesto sauce
- 1/4 cup cherry tomatoes, halved
- 1 tablespoon olive oil
- Salt and pepper to taste

Directions:

1. Heat olive oil in a skillet over medium heat.
2. Add zucchini noodles and cook until slightly tender.
3. Remove from heat and toss with pesto sauce and cherry tomatoes.
4. Season with salt and pepper and serve.

Serving:

2 servings

Nutrition (per serving):

Calories: 200

Carbohydrates: 8g

Protein: 4g

Fat: 18g

3. Tuna Salad Lettuce Wraps

Ingredients:

- 1 can tuna, drained
- 1/4 cup mayonnaise
- 1 celery stalk, diced
- 1 tablespoon lemon juice
- 1/2 avocado, diced
- Salt and pepper to taste
- Large lettuce leaves for wrapping

Directions:

1. In a bowl, combine tuna, mayonnaise, celery, lemon juice, avocado, salt, and pepper.

2. Mix well.

3. Spoon tuna salad onto lettuce leaves and wrap.

4. Serve immediately.

Serving:

2 servings

Nutrition (per serving):

Calories: 250

Carbohydrates: 4g

Protein: 20g

Fat: 18g

4. Egg Salad with Avocado

Ingredients:

- 3 hard-boiled eggs, chopped
- 1/2 avocado, diced
- 2 tablespoons mayonnaise
- 1 teaspoon Dijon mustard
- 1 tablespoon lemon juice
- Salt and pepper to taste

Directions:

1. In a bowl, combine chopped eggs, avocado, mayonnaise, Dijon mustard, lemon juice, salt, and pepper.

2. Mix well.

3. Serve immediately.

Serving:

1 serving
Nutrition:

Calories: 300
Carbohydrates: 6g
Protein: 15g
Fat: 24g

5. Beef and Broccoli Stir-Fry
Ingredients:

- 1 cup broccoli florets
- 1/2 cup sliced beef (sirloin or flank steak)
- 1 tablespoon soy sauce
- 1 tablespoon sesame oil
- 1 garlic clove, minced
- 1/2 teaspoon ginger, minced
- Salt and pepper to taste

Directions:

- Heat sesame oil in a skillet over medium heat.
- Add garlic and ginger and cook until fragrant.
- Add beef and cook until browned.
- Add broccoli and soy sauce.
- Cook until broccoli is tender.
- Season with salt and pepper and serve.

Serving:

1 serving
Nutrition:

Calories: 250

Carbohydrates: 10g

Protein: 20g

Fat: 15g

6. Cauliflower Fried Rice

Ingredients:

- 2 cups riced cauliflower
- 1/2 cup mixed vegetables (carrots, peas)
- 1 egg, beaten
- 1 tablespoon soy sauce
- 1 tablespoon sesame oil
- 1 garlic clove, minced
- Salt and pepper to taste

Directions:

- Heat sesame oil in a skillet over medium heat.
- Add garlic and cook until fragrant.
- Add mixed vegetables and cook until tender.
- Add riced cauliflower and soy sauce.
- Push the mixture to the side of the skillet and pour the beaten egg into the empty space.
- Scramble the egg, then mix it into the cauliflower rice.
- Season with salt and pepper and serve.

Serving:

2 servings
Nutrition (per serving):

Calories: 150
Carbohydrates: 10g
Protein: 6g
Fat: 10g

7. Turkey and Avocado Roll-Ups
Ingredients:

- 4 slices turkey breast
- 1/2 avocado, sliced
- 4 slices cucumber
- 1/4 cup sprouts

Directions:

1. Lay turkey slices flat.
2. Place avocado slices, cucumber slices, and sprouts on each slice.
3. Roll up the turkey slices around the fillings.
4. Serve immediately.

Serving:

1 serving
Nutrition:

Calories: 200

Carbohydrates: 6g

Protein: 18g

Fat: 12g

7.3 Dinner Recipes

High-Carb Dinner Recipes

1. Baked Salmon with Quinoa and Veggies

Ingredients:

- 2 salmon fillets
- 1 cup cooked quinoa
- 1 cup broccoli florets
- 1 cup cherry tomatoes, halved
- 1 tablespoon olive oil
- 1 lemon, sliced
- Salt and pepper to taste

Directions:

1. Preheat oven to 400°F (200°C).
2. Place salmon fillets on a baking sheet, drizzle with olive oil, and season with salt and pepper. Top with lemon slices.
3. Bake for 15-20 minutes or until salmon is cooked through.
4. While salmon is baking, steam broccoli until tender.
5. Serve salmon with quinoa and steamed broccoli, and top with cherry tomatoes.

Serving:

2 servings

Nutrition (per serving):

Calories: 450
Carbohydrates: 35g

Protein: 40g

Fat: 15g

2. Chickpea and Spinach Curry

Ingredients:

- 1 can chickpeas, drained and rinsed
- 2 cups spinach leaves
- 1 cup diced tomatoes
- 1 onion, diced
- 2 garlic cloves, minced
- 1 tablespoon curry powder
- 1 tablespoon olive oil
- 1 cup brown rice, cooked
- Salt and pepper to taste

Directions:

1. Heat olive oil in a skillet over medium heat.
2. Add onion and garlic and sauté until translucent.
3. Add curry powder and cook for another minute.
4. Add diced tomatoes and chickpeas, and cook until heated through.
5. Stir in spinach and cook until wilted.
6. Serve curry over cooked brown rice.

Serving:

2 servings

Nutrition (per serving):

Calories: 400

Carbohydrates: 65g

Protein: 15g

Fat: 10g

3. Whole Wheat Spaghetti with Marinara Sauce

Ingredients:

- 2 cups cooked whole wheat spaghetti
- 1 cup marinara sauce
- 1 zucchini, sliced
- 1 bell pepper, diced
- 1/4 cup grated Parmesan cheese
- 1 tablespoon olive oil
- Salt and pepper to taste

Directions:

1. Heat olive oil in a skillet over medium heat.
2. Add zucchini and bell pepper and cook until tender.
3. Add marinara sauce and cook until heated through.
4. Toss the sauce with cooked spaghetti.
5. Sprinkle with Parmesan cheese and serve.

Serving:

2 servings

Nutrition (per serving):

Calories: 350

Carbohydrates: 60g

Protein: 12g

Fat: 10g

4. Black Bean and Corn Tacos

Ingredients:

- 1 cup black beans, drained and rinsed
- 1/2 cup corn kernels
- 1/4 cup red onion, diced
- 1/4 cup cilantro, chopped
- 1/4 cup salsa
- 1 avocado, sliced
- 4 whole wheat tortillas

Directions:

1. In a bowl, combine black beans, corn, red onion, and cilantro.
2. Heat tortillas in a skillet or microwave.
3. Divide the black bean mixture among the tortillas.
4. Top with salsa and avocado slices.
5. Serve immediately.

Serving:

2 servings

Nutrition (per serving):

Calories: 400

Carbohydrates: 55g

Protein: 12g

Fat: 15g

5. Lentil and Sweet Potato Stew

Ingredients:

- 1 cup lentils, rinsed
- 1 sweet potato, peeled and diced
- 1 carrot, diced
- 1 celery stalk, diced
- 1 onion, diced
- 2 cups vegetable broth
- 1 cup diced tomatoes
- 1 teaspoon cumin
- 1 teaspoon paprika
- Salt and pepper to taste

Directions:

1. In a large pot, combine lentils, sweet potato, carrot, celery, onion, and vegetable broth.
2. Bring to a boil, then reduce heat and simmer until lentils are tender.
3. Add diced tomatoes, cumin, paprika, salt, and pepper.
4. Simmer for another 10 minutes and serve.

Serving:

2 servings

Nutrition (per serving):

Calories: 350
Carbohydrates: 60g
Protein: 15g
Fat: 2g

6. Chicken and Brown Rice Stir-Fry

Ingredients:

- 1 cup cooked brown rice
- 1 cup diced chicken breast
- 1 cup mixed vegetables (broccoli, bell pepper, carrots)
- 2 tablespoons soy sauce
- 1 tablespoon sesame oil
- 1 garlic clove, minced

Directions:

1. Heat sesame oil in a skillet over medium heat.
2. Add garlic and cook until fragrant.
3. Add chicken and cook until browned.
4. Add mixed vegetables and cook until tender.
5. Add cooked brown rice and soy sauce.
6. Toss to combine and serve.

Serving:

2 servings

Nutrition (per serving):

Calories: 450

Carbohydrates: 50g

Protein: 30g

Fat: 12g

7. Sweet Potato and Black Bean Enchiladas

Ingredients:

- 2 large sweet potatoes, peeled and diced
- 1 can black beans, drained and rinsed
- 1 cup enchilada sauce
- 1/2 cup shredded cheese
- 4 whole wheat tortillas
- 1/4 cup chopped cilantro

Directions:

1. Preheat oven to 375°F (190°C).
2. Cook sweet potatoes in a skillet over medium heat until tender.
3. Add black beans and cook until heated through.
4. Fill tortillas with sweet potato and black bean mixture, and roll up.
5. Place enchiladas in a baking dish and cover with enchilada sauce.
6. Sprinkle with cheese and bake for 20 minutes or until cheese is melted.
7. Garnish with chopped cilantro and serve.

Serving:

2 servings

Nutrition (per serving):

Calories: 500

Carbohydrates: 80g

Protein: 20g

Fat: 12g

Low-Carb Dinner Recipes

1. Grilled Chicken with Asparagus

Ingredients:

- 2 chicken breasts
- 1 bunch asparagus, trimmed
- 2 tablespoons olive oil
- 1 tablespoon lemon juice
- Salt and pepper to taste

Directions:

1. Preheat grill to medium-high heat.
2. Drizzle chicken breasts and asparagus with olive oil and lemon juice.
3. Season with salt and pepper.
4. Grill chicken for 5-7 minutes on each side or until cooked through.
5. Grill asparagus for 2-3 minutes on each side.
6. Serve chicken with asparagus.

Serving:

2 servings

Nutrition (per serving):

Calories: 300

Carbohydrates: 5g

Protein: 30g

Fat: 15g

2. Zucchini Lasagna

Ingredients:

- 2 large zucchinis, sliced lengthwise
- 1 cup marinara sauce
- 1 cup ricotta cheese
- 1/2 cup shredded mozzarella cheese
- 1/4 cup grated Parmesan cheese
- 1 egg
- 1 teaspoon Italian seasoning
- Salt and pepper to taste

Directions:

1. Preheat oven to 375°F (190°C).
2. In a bowl, mix ricotta cheese, egg, Italian seasoning, salt, and pepper.
3. Layer zucchini slices, ricotta mixture, and marinara sauce in a baking dish.
4. Repeat layers until all ingredients are used.
5. Top with mozzarella and Parmesan cheese.
6. Bake for 25-30 minutes or until cheese is bubbly and golden.
7. Serve immediately.

Serving:

2 servings

Nutrition (per serving):

Calories: 350

Carbohydrates: 10g

Protein: 25g

Fat: 20g

3. Baked Cod with Spinach and Tomatoes

Ingredients:

- 2 cod fillets
- 2 cups spinach leaves
- 1 cup cherry tomatoes, halved
- 2 tablespoons olive oil
- 1 lemon, sliced
- Salt and pepper to taste

Directions:

- Preheat oven to 400°F (200°C).
- Place cod fillets in a baking dish, drizzle with olive oil, and season with salt and pepper. Top with lemon slices.
- Bake for 15-20 minutes or until cod is cooked through.
- In a skillet, sauté spinach and cherry tomatoes in olive oil until spinach is wilted.
- Serve cod with spinach and tomatoes.

Serving:

2 servings

Nutrition (per serving):

Calories: 250

Carbohydrates: 6g

Protein: 25g

Fat: 14g

4. Grilled Steak with Roasted Vegetables

Ingredients:

- 2 steaks (your choice of cut)
- 1 bell pepper, sliced
- 1 zucchini, sliced
- 1 onion, sliced
- 2 tablespoons olive oil
- Salt and pepper to taste

Directions:

1. Preheat grill to medium-high heat.
2. Toss vegetables with olive oil, salt, and pepper.
3. Grill steaks for 4-5 minutes on each side for medium-rare, or to desired doneness.
4. Grill vegetables for 5-7 minutes until tender.
5. Serve steaks with roasted vegetables.

Serving:

2 servings

Nutrition (per serving):

Calories: 400

Carbohydrates: 10g

Protein: 35g

Fat: 25g

5. Spinach and Mushroom Stuffed Chicken Breast

Ingredients:

- 2 chicken breasts

- 1 cup spinach, chopped
- 1/2 cup mushrooms, sliced
- 1/4 cup feta cheese, crumbled
- 1 garlic clove, minced
- 1 tablespoon olive oil
- Salt and pepper to taste

Directions:

1. Preheat oven to 375°F (190°C).
2. In a skillet, heat olive oil over medium heat.
3. Add garlic and cook until fragrant.
4. Add spinach and mushrooms, and cook until spinach is wilted and mushrooms are tender.
5. Stir in feta cheese, salt, and pepper.
6. Cut a pocket into each chicken breast and stuff with spinach mixture.
7. Bake for 25-30 minutes or until chicken is cooked through.
8. Serve immediately.

Serving:

2 servings

Nutrition (per serving):

Calories: 300

Carbohydrates: 5g

Protein: 35g

Fat: 15g

6. Shrimp and Avocado Salad

Ingredients:

- 1 lb shrimp, peeled and deveined
- 2 avocados, diced
- 2 cups mixed greens
- 1/2 cup cherry tomatoes, halved
- 1/4 cup red onion, thinly sliced
- 2 tablespoons olive oil
- 1 tablespoon balsamic vinegar
- Salt and pepper to taste

Directions:

- Heat olive oil in a skillet over medium heat.
- Add shrimp and cook for 2-3 minutes per side until pink and cooked through.
- In a large bowl, toss mixed greens, cherry tomatoes, red onion, avocado, cooked shrimp, olive oil, and balsamic vinegar.
- Season with salt and pepper.
- Serve immediately.

Serving:

2 servings

Nutrition (per serving):

Calories: 350

Carbohydrates: 10g

Protein: 30g

Fat: 20g

7.4 Snacks and Smoothies

High-Carb Snacks and Smoothies

1. Banana and Peanut Butter Smoothie
Ingredients:

- 1 banana
- 2 tablespoons peanut butter
- 1 cup milk (or almond milk for a dairy-free option)
- 1 tablespoon honey (optional)
- Ice cubes

Directions:

1. Blend banana, peanut butter, milk, and honey until smooth.
2. Add ice cubes and blend again until desired consistency is reached.
3. Serve immediately.

Serving: Makes 1 serving

Nutrition (per serving):

Calories: 350
Carbohydrates: 40g
Protein: 10g
Fat: 18g

2. Greek Yogurt with Berries

Ingredients:

- 1 cup Greek yogurt
- 1/2 cup mixed berries (strawberries, blueberries, raspberries)
- 1 tablespoon honey (optional)
- 1 tablespoon chopped nuts (almonds, walnuts)

Directions:

1. Spoon Greek yogurt into a bowl.
2. Top with mixed berries.
3. Drizzle with honey and sprinkle with chopped nuts.

Serving: Makes 1 serving

Nutrition (per serving):

Calories: 250

Carbohydrates: 30g

Protein: 20g

Fat: 8g

3. Apple Slices with Almond Butter

Ingredients:

- 1 apple, sliced
- 2 tablespoons almond butter
- Cinnamon (optional)

Directions:

1. Spread almond butter on apple slices.

2. Sprinkle with cinnamon if desired.
3. Serve immediately.

Serving: Makes 1 serving

Nutrition (per serving):

Calories: 200
Carbohydrates: 25g
Protein: 5g
Fat: 10g

4. Oatmeal with Fruit

Ingredients:

- 1/2 cup rolled oats
- 1 cup milk (or water)
- 1/2 cup mixed fruit (banana slices, berries)
- 1 tablespoon honey or maple syrup
- Cinnamon (optional)

Directions:

1. Cook rolled oats with milk or water according to package instructions.
2. Top with mixed fruit.
3. Drizzle with honey or maple syrup and sprinkle with cinnamon if desired.
4. Serve warm.

Serving: Makes 1 serving

Nutrition (per serving):

Calories: 300

Carbohydrates: 50g

Protein: 8g

Fat: 7g

5. Mango and Pineapple Smoothie

Ingredients:

- 1 cup mango chunks
- 1/2 cup pineapple chunks
- 1/2 cup plain yogurt (or coconut yogurt for a dairy-free option)
- 1/2 cup orange juice
- Ice cubes

Directions:

1. Blend mango, pineapple, yogurt, and orange juice until smooth.
2. Add ice cubes and blend again until desired consistency is reached.
3. Serve immediately.

Serving: Makes 1 serving

Nutrition (per serving):

Calories: 300

Carbohydrates: 70g

Protein: 6g

Fat: 2g

6. Rice Cakes with Jam

Ingredients:

- 2 rice cakes
- 2 tablespoons fruit jam (choose a variety without added sugar)

Directions:

1. Spread jam on rice cakes.
2. Serve immediately.

Serving: Makes 1 serving

Nutrition (per serving):

Calories: 150
Carbohydrates: 35g
Protein: 1g
Fat: 0g

7. Energy Balls

Ingredients:

- 1 cup rolled oats
- 1/2 cup peanut butter
- 1/4 cup honey
- 1/4 cup chocolate chips (optional)
- 1/4 cup dried fruit (raisins, cranberries)

Directions:

1. Mix rolled oats, peanut butter, honey, chocolate chips, and dried fruit in a bowl until well combined.

2. Roll into small balls using your hands.

3. Refrigerate for 30 minutes to set.

4. Serve chilled.

Serving: Makes 12 balls

Nutrition (per serving, 1 ball):

Calories: 150

Carbohydrates: 18g

Protein: 4g

Fat: 8g

Low-Carb Snacks and Smoothies

1. Avocado with Cottage Cheese

Ingredients:

- 1 avocado, sliced
- 1/2 cup cottage cheese
- Salt and pepper to taste

Directions:

1. Top avocado slices with cottage cheese.

2. Season with salt and pepper.

3. Serve immediately.

Serving: Makes 1 serving

Nutrition (per serving):

Calories: 250

Carbohydrates: 10g

Protein: 15g

Fat: 18g

2. Cucumber Slices with Hummus

Ingredients:

- 1 cucumber, sliced
- 1/4 cup hummus

Directions:

1. Serve cucumber slices with hummus for dipping.
2. Serve immediately.

Serving: Makes 1 serving

Nutrition (per serving):

Calories: 150

Carbohydrates: 15g

Protein: 5g

Fat: 8g

3. Cheese and Pepperoni Slices

Ingredients:

- 1 oz cheese (cheddar, mozzarella)
- 1 oz pepperoni slices

Directions:

1. Arrange cheese and pepperoni slices on a plate.

2. Serve immediately.

Serving: Makes 1 serving

Nutrition (per serving):

Calories: 250
Carbohydrates: 2g
Protein: 15g
Fat: 20g

4. Almonds and Berries

Ingredients:

- 1/4 cup almonds
- 1/2 cup mixed berries (strawberries, blueberries)

Directions:

1. Serve almonds with mixed berries.
2. Serve immediately.

Serving: Makes 1 serving

Nutrition (per serving):

Calories: 200
Carbohydrates: 15g
Protein: 6g
Fat: 14g

5. Egg Salad Lettuce Wraps

Ingredients:

- 2 hard-boiled eggs, chopped
- 1 tablespoon mayonnaise
- 1 teaspoon mustard
- Salt and pepper to taste
- Lettuce leaves for wrapping

Directions:

1. Mix chopped eggs, mayonnaise, mustard, salt, and pepper in a bowl until well combined.
2. Spoon egg salad onto lettuce leaves.
3. Wrap and serve immediately.

Serving: Makes 1 serving

Nutrition (per serving):

Calories: 250

Carbohydrates: 3g

Protein: 12g

Fat: 20g

6. Celery Sticks with Cream Cheese

Ingredients:

- 2 celery stalks, cut into sticks
- 2 tablespoons cream cheese

Directions:

1. Spread cream cheese on celery sticks.
2. Serve immediately.

Serving: Makes 1 serving

Nutrition (per serving):

Calories: 150
Carbohydrates: 5g
Protein: 3g
Fat: 12g

7. Green Smoothie

Ingredients:

- 1 cup spinach
- 1/2 avocado
- 1/2 cucumber
- 1/2 cup almond milk
- Juice of 1/2 lemon
- Ice cubes

Directions:

1. Blend spinach, avocado, cucumber, almond milk, and lemon juice until smooth.
2. Add ice cubes and blend again until desired consistency is reached.
3. Serve immediately.

Serving: Makes 1 serving

Nutrition (per serving):

Calories: 200
Carbohydrates: 10g
Protein: 5g
Fat: 15g

7.5 Desserts

High-Carb Desserts

1. Fruit Salad with Yogurt
Ingredients:

- 1 cup mixed fruit (strawberries, kiwi, pineapple)
- 1/2 cup Greek yogurt
- 1 tablespoon honey (optional)

Directions:

- Chop fruit into bite-sized pieces and mix in a bowl.
- Serve with Greek yogurt drizzled with honey.

Serving: Makes 1 serving

Nutrition (per serving):

Calories: 200
Carbohydrates: 40g
Protein: 10g
Fat: 2g

2. Berry Parfait
Ingredients:

- 1 cup mixed berries (strawberries, blueberries, raspberries)
- 1 cup Greek yogurt
- 1/4 cup granola

Directions:

1. Layer Greek yogurt, mixed berries, and granola in a glass or bowl.
2. Repeat layers as desired.
3. Serve chilled.

Serving: Makes 1 serving

Nutrition (per serving):

Calories: 300

Carbohydrates: 45g

Protein: 15g

Fat: 6g

3. Banana Bread

Ingredients:

- 2 ripe bananas, mashed
- 1/4 cup melted butter
- 1/2 cup sugar
- 1 egg, beaten
- 1 teaspoon vanilla extract
- 1 teaspoon baking soda
- Pinch of salt
- 1 1/2 cups all-purpose flour

Directions:

1. Preheat oven to 350°F (175°C). Grease a 4x8 inch loaf pan.
2. In a mixing bowl, combine mashed bananas, melted butter, sugar, egg, and vanilla extract.

3. Mix in baking soda and salt.

4. Add flour and mix until smooth.

5. Pour batter into prepared loaf pan.

6. Bake for 60-65 minutes or until a toothpick inserted into the center comes out clean.

7. Allow to cool before slicing and serving.

Serving: Makes 10 servings

Nutrition (per serving):

Calories: 250

Carbohydrates: 40g

Protein: 3g

Fat: 9g

4. Rice Pudding

Ingredients:

- 1/2 cup rice (jasmine or basmati)
- 2 cups milk (or coconut milk for a dairy-free option)
- 1/4 cup sugar
- 1 teaspoon vanilla extract
- Cinnamon (optional)

Directions:

1. Rinse rice under cold water.

2. In a saucepan, bring milk and rice to a boil. Reduce heat, cover, and simmer for 20-25 minutes or until rice is tender.

3. Stir in sugar and vanilla extract.

4. Cook uncovered over medium heat for 5-10 minutes until thickened.

5. Remove from heat and let cool.

6. Sprinkle with cinnamon if desired before serving.

Serving: Makes 4 servings

Nutrition (per serving):

Calories: 300

Carbohydrates: 50g

Protein: 6g

Fat: 8g

5. Chocolate Chip Cookies

Ingredients:

- 1/2 cup butter, softened
- 1/2 cup white sugar
- 1/2 cup packed brown sugar
- 1 egg
- 1 teaspoon vanilla extract
- 1 1/2 cups all-purpose flour
- 1/2 teaspoon baking soda
- 1/2 teaspoon salt
- 1 cup semisweet chocolate chips

Directions:

1. Preheat oven to 350°F (175°C). Grease cookie sheets.
2. In a large bowl, cream together butter, white sugar, and brown sugar until smooth.
3. Beat in egg and vanilla extract.
4. Combine flour, baking soda, and salt; gradually stir into the creamed mixture.

5. Mix in chocolate chips.

6. Drop rounded spoonfuls onto prepared cookie sheets.

7. Bake for 10-12 minutes or until edges are golden brown.

8. Allow cookies to cool on baking sheet for 5 minutes before transferring to wire racks to cool completely.

Serving: Makes 24 cookies

Nutrition (per cookie):

Calories: 150

Carbohydrates: 20g

Protein: 2g

Fat: 7g

6. Apple Crisp

Ingredients:

- 4 cups sliced apples
- 1 tablespoon lemon juice
- 1/2 cup rolled oats
- 1/2 cup all-purpose flour
- 1/2 cup packed brown sugar
- 1/4 cup butter, softened
- 1/2 teaspoon ground cinnamon
- 1/4 teaspoon ground nutmeg

Directions:

1. Preheat oven to 350°F (175°C). Grease a 9-inch square baking dish.

2. Place sliced apples in the prepared baking dish and sprinkle with lemon juice.

3. In a separate bowl, combine rolled oats, flour, brown sugar, butter, cinnamon, and nutmeg until crumbly.

4. Sprinkle oat mixture evenly over apples.

5. Bake for 40-45 minutes or until apples are tender and topping is golden brown.

6. Serve warm.

Serving: Makes 6 servings

Nutrition (per serving):

Calories: 300

Carbohydrates: 50g

Protein: 2g

Fat: 10g

7. Mango Sorbet

Ingredients:

- 2 ripe mangoes, peeled and diced
- 1/4 cup sugar
- Juice of 1 lime
- 1/4 cup water

Directions:

1. In a blender, combine diced mangoes, sugar, lime juice, and water.

2. Blend until smooth.

3. Pour mixture into a shallow dish and freeze for 4 hours or until firm.

4. Scrape with a fork to create a fluffy texture.

5. Serve immediately.

Serving: Makes 4 servings

Nutrition (per serving):

Calories: 150
Carbohydrates: 35g
Protein: 1g
Fat: 0g

Low-Carb Desserts

1. Chocolate Avocado Mousse
Ingredients:

- 2 ripe avocados, peeled and pitted
- 1/4 cup cocoa powder
- 1/4 cup almond milk
- 1/4 cup sugar-free sweetener (erythritol or stevia)
- 1 teaspoon vanilla extract

Directions:

1. In a blender or food processor, blend avocados, cocoa powder, almond milk, sweetener, and vanilla extract until smooth and creamy.
2. Chill in the refrigerator for 30 minutes before serving.

Serving: Makes 4 servings

Nutrition (per serving):

Calories: 200
Carbohydrates: 12g
Protein: 3g
Fat: 15g

2. Chia Seed Pudding

Ingredients:

- 1/4 cup chia seeds
- 1 cup almond milk
- 1 tablespoon sugar-free sweetener (erythritol or stevia)
- 1/2 teaspoon vanilla extract
- Berries for topping

Directions:

1. In a bowl, mix chia seeds, almond milk, sweetener, and vanilla extract.
2. Cover and refrigerate for at least 2 hours or overnight until thickened.
3. Stir well before serving and top with berries.

Serving: Makes 2 servings

Nutrition (per serving):

Calories: 150

Carbohydrates: 10g

Protein: 5g

Fat: 9g

3. Peanut Butter Cookies

Ingredients:

- 1 cup peanut butter
- 1/2 cup sugar-free sweetener (erythritol or stevia)
- 1 egg
- 1 teaspoon vanilla extract

Directions:

1. Preheat oven to 350°F (175°C). Line a baking sheet with parchment paper.
2. In a bowl, mix peanut butter, sweetener, egg, and vanilla extract until well combined.
3. Scoop tablespoon-sized balls of dough onto the prepared baking sheet.
4. Flatten each ball with a fork, making a crisscross pattern.
5. Bake for 10-12 minutes or until edges are golden brown.
6. Allow cookies to cool on baking sheet for 5 minutes before transferring to wire racks to cool completely.

Serving: Makes 12 cookies

Nutrition (per cookie):

Calories: 150
Carbohydrates: 5g
Protein: 6g
Fat: 12g

4. Coconut Flour Pancakes

Ingredients:

1/4 cup coconut flour
1/4 teaspoon baking powder
2 eggs
1/4 cup almond milk
1 tablespoon coconut oil, melted
Sugar-free syrup (optional)

Directions:

1. In a bowl, whisk together coconut flour and baking powder.
2. In another bowl, whisk eggs, almond milk, and melted coconut oil.
3. Add wet ingredients to dry ingredients and mix until smooth.
4. Heat a non-stick skillet over medium heat and lightly grease with coconut oil.
5. Pour 1/4 cup of batter onto the skillet for each pancake.
6. Cook for 2-3 minutes on each side or until golden brown.
7. Serve with sugar-free syrup if desired.

Serving: Makes 2 servings (4 pancakes)

Nutrition (per serving):

Calories: 200
Carbohydrates: 10g
Protein: 8g
Fat: 15g

5. Avocado Chocolate Pudding

Ingredients:

- 2 ripe avocados, peeled and pitted
- 1/4 cup cocoa powder
- 1/4 cup sugar-free sweetener (erythritol or stevia)
- 1/4 cup almond milk
- 1 teaspoon vanilla extract

Directions:

1. In a blender or food processor, blend avocados, cocoa powder, sweetener, almond milk, and vanilla extract until smooth.

2. Chill in the refrigerator for 30 minutes before serving.

Serving: Makes 4 servings

Nutrition (per serving):

Calories: 150

Carbohydrates: 10g

Protein: 3g

Fat: 12g

6. Lemon Cheesecake Fat Bombs

Ingredients:

- 1/2 cup cream cheese, softened
- 2 tablespoons butter, softened
- 1 tablespoon lemon juice
- Zest of 1 lemon
- 1/4 cup sugar-free sweetener (erythritol or stevia)

Directions:

1. In a bowl, combine cream cheese, butter, lemon juice, lemon zest, and sweetener until smooth.
2. Spoon mixture into mini muffin cups lined with paper liners.
3. Freeze for 1-2 hours until firm.
4. Remove from muffin cups and serve chilled.

Serving: Makes 6 fat bombs

Nutrition (per fat bomb):

Calories: 100

Carbohydrates: 2g

Protein: 2g

Fat: 10g

7. Mixed Berry Sorbet

Ingredients:

- 2 cups mixed berries (strawberries, blueberries, raspberries)
- Juice of 1/2 lemon
- 1/4 cup water
- 1/4 cup sugar-free sweetener (erythritol or stevia)

Directions:

1. In a blender, combine mixed berries, lemon juice, water, and sweetener until smooth.
2. Pour mixture into a shallow dish and freeze for 4 hours or until firm.
3. Scrape with a fork to create a fluffy texture.
4. Serve immediately.

Serving: Makes 4 servings

Nutrition (per serving):

Calories: 50

Carbohydrates: 10g

Protein: 1g

Fat: 1g

Chapter 8: Exercise and Carb Cycling

8.1 Importance of Exercise for Women Over 50

Exercise is crucial for women over 50 as it plays a pivotal role in maintaining overall health, mobility, and quality of life during this stage of life. Here's why exercise is particularly important for women in this age group:

1. Maintaining Muscle Mass and Strength: As women age, they naturally lose muscle mass and strength. Regular exercise, especially resistance training, helps to preserve muscle tissue, improve strength, and enhance overall physical function. This is vital for maintaining independence and reducing the risk of falls and fractures.

2. Bone Health: Post-menopause, women are at a higher risk of osteoporosis and bone fractures due to decreased estrogen levels. Weight-bearing exercises such as walking, jogging, dancing, and strength training help to maintain bone density and reduce the risk of osteoporosis.

3. Heart Health: Cardiovascular health becomes increasingly important with age. Regular aerobic exercise, such as brisk walking, swimming, or cycling, helps to improve heart function, lower blood pressure, and reduce the risk of heart disease and stroke.

4. Weight Management: Metabolism tends to slow down with age, making weight management more challenging. Exercise, along with a balanced diet, helps to maintain a healthy weight by burning calories, preserving lean muscle mass, and boosting metabolism.

5. Joint Health and Flexibility: Regular physical activity improves joint flexibility and mobility, reducing stiffness and joint pain. Activities like yoga, tai chi, and stretching exercises are particularly beneficial for maintaining flexibility and range of motion.

6. Mental Well-being: Exercise has significant mental health benefits, including reducing stress, anxiety, and depression. Physical activity stimulates the production of endorphins, which are natural mood lifters, promoting a sense of well-being and improving sleep quality.

7. Improving Balance and Coordination: Balance and coordination tend to decline with age, increasing the risk of falls. Exercises that challenge balance, such as yoga, tai chi, and specific balance drills, help to improve stability and reduce the risk of falls.

8. Social Engagement: Participating in group exercise classes or activities can provide social interaction and support, reducing feelings of loneliness and isolation that may occur as women age.

9. Longevity and Quality of Life: Engaging in regular exercise is associated with increased longevity and improved overall quality of life. It enhances energy levels, cognitive function, and overall physical capabilities, allowing women to maintain an active and independent lifestyle.

For women over 50, it's essential to incorporate a variety of exercises that address strength, cardiovascular fitness, flexibility, and balance into their weekly routine. Consulting with a healthcare provider or a certified fitness professional can help tailor an exercise program that meets individual needs and goals while ensuring safety and effectiveness.

8.2 Best Types of Exercise to Complement Carb Cycling

Certainly! When complimenting carb cycling with exercise, it's essential to choose activities that support your energy needs and metabolic goals. Here are some of the best types of exercises to consider:

1. Strength Training: Incorporating resistance exercises such as weight lifting or bodyweight exercises helps to build and maintain lean muscle mass. This is particularly beneficial during high-carb days when muscles can utilize carbohydrates for energy and recovery.

2. High-Intensity Interval Training (HIIT): HIIT exercises include short eruptions of serious activity followed by times of rest or lower force. These workouts can be effective during both high-carb and low-carb days, as they improve cardiovascular fitness, boost metabolism, and enhance fat burning.

3. Circuit Training: Circuit training combines strength exercises with aerobic activities in a series of stations or intervals. It's a versatile workout that can be adjusted based on carb cycling phases to maximize muscle glycogen storage during high-carb days and fat utilization during low-carb days.

4. Aerobic Exercise: Activities like walking, jogging, cycling, or swimming provide cardiovascular benefits and can be tailored to fit different carb cycling phases. During high-carb days, aerobic exercise helps to utilize carbohydrates for energy, while during low-carb days, it enhances fat oxidation.

5. Yoga and Pilates: These exercises focus on flexibility, balance, and core strength. They are excellent choices for recovery days or during low-carb phases, as they promote relaxation, improve mobility, and support overall well-being.

6. Sports and Recreational Activities: Engaging in sports such as tennis, basketball, or hiking can provide both aerobic and anaerobic benefits. These activities can be enjoyable additions to high-carb days when energy levels are higher.

7. Flexibility and Mobility Work: Including stretching exercises, foam rolling, or mobility drills helps to maintain joint health and prevent stiffness. These exercises can be beneficial throughout the carb cycling cycle to enhance recovery and overall flexibility.

8. Mind-Body Exercises: Practices such as tai chi or qigong combine movement, meditation, and deep breathing. They promote relaxation, reduce stress, and complement the holistic approach of carb cycling by supporting mental well-being and overall balance.

When incorporating exercise into your carb cycling plan, it's essential to listen to your body, adjust the intensity based on energy levels, and stay hydrated. Consult with a fitness professional or healthcare provider to create a personalized exercise regimen that aligns with your carb cycling goals and overall health objectives.

8.3 Sample Workout Plans

Day 1: High-Carb Day
- **Warm-Up:** 5-10 minutes of dynamic stretching or light cardio.

Strength Training:
- Squats: 3 sets of 12 reps
- Bench Press (or push-ups): 3 sets of 12 reps
- Bent-over Rows: 3 sets of 12 reps

Cardio: 20 minutes of moderate-intensity cardio (e.g., jogging, cycling).

Cool Down: 5-10 minutes of static stretching.

Day 2: Low-Carb Day
- **Warm-Up:** 5-10 minutes of dynamic stretching or light cardio.
- **HIIT Workout:** 15 minutes of high-intensity interval training (e.g., 30 seconds sprinting followed by 1 minute walking/jogging).

Strength Training:
- Lunges: 3 sets of 12 reps per leg
- Push-ups (or incline push-ups): 3 sets of 12 reps
- Plank with Shoulder Taps: 3 sets of 30 seconds

Cool Down: 5-10 minutes of static stretching and deep breathing exercises.

Day 3: High-Carb Day

Warm-Up: 5-10 minutes of dynamic stretching or light cardio.

Upper Body Strength Training:
- Shoulder Press: 3 sets of 12 reps
- Pull-ups (or assisted pull-ups): 3 sets of 8-10 reps
- Bicep Curls: 3 sets of 12 reps

Cardio: 15 minutes of moderate-intensity cardio (e.g., rowing, elliptical).

Cool Down: 5-10 minutes of static stretching focusing on upper body muscles.

Day 4: Low-Carb Day

Warm-Up: 5-10 minutes of dynamic stretching or light cardio.

Lower Body Strength Training:

- Deadlifts (or Romanian deadlifts): 3 sets of 12 reps
- Bodyweight Squats: 3 sets of 15 reps
- Calf Raises: 3 sets of 15 reps

HIIT Workout: 20 minutes of alternating between 30 seconds of high-intensity exercise (e.g., sprinting, jumping jacks) and 1 minute of low-intensity exercise (e.g., walking).

Cool Down: 5-10 minutes of static stretching focusing on lower body muscles.

Day 5: High-Carb Day

Warm-Up: 5-10 minutes of dynamic stretching or light cardio.

Full-Body Circuit:

- Step-ups: 3 sets of 15 reps per leg
- Dips (or chair dips): 3 sets of 12 reps
- Plank: 3 sets of 30 seconds

Cardio: 20 minutes of moderate-intensity cardio (e.g., brisk walking, cycling).

Cool Down: 5-10 minutes of static stretching.

Day 6: Low-Carb Day

Warm-Up: 5-10 minutes of dynamic stretching or light cardio.

HIIT Workout: 15 minutes of high-intensity interval training (e.g., 30 seconds sprinting followed by 1 minute walking/jogging).

Strength Training:

- Push-ups (or modified push-ups): 3 sets of 15 reps
- Bodyweight Lunges: 3 sets of 15 reps per leg
- Plank with Leg Lifts: 3 sets of 30 seconds

Cool Down: 5-10 minutes of static stretching and deep breathing exercises.

Day 7: Active Recovery

Activities:

- Gentle Yoga or Stretching: 20-30 minutes to promote flexibility and relaxation.
- Walking or Light Cycling: 30-45 minutes of low-intensity activity to improve circulation and aid in recovery.

Focus: Enhance recovery and prepare for the upcoming week's workouts.

8.4 Stretching and Recovery

Stretching and recovery are essential components of any exercise program, particularly when complimenting carb cycling. They help improve flexibility, reduce muscle tension, and enhance overall recovery. Here's why stretching and recovery are crucial:

1. Flexibility Enhancement: Regular stretching improves flexibility by lengthening muscles and increasing range of motion. This is beneficial for maintaining joint health and preventing injuries, especially during intense workouts.

2. Muscle Recovery: Stretching promotes blood flow to muscles, which aids in the delivery of nutrients and removal of waste products. This accelerates muscle recovery and reduces soreness after workouts.

3. Relaxation and Stress Reduction: Stretching exercises, particularly those involving deep breathing and gentle movements (e.g., yoga), promote relaxation and reduce stress levels. This contributes to overall well-being and supports mental clarity.

4. Improved Performance: Incorporating stretching into your routine can enhance athletic performance by preparing muscles for exercise, improving muscle coordination, and optimizing movement patterns.

5. Injury Prevention: Flexible muscles and tendons are less prone to strains and sprains. Stretching before and after workouts helps maintain muscle elasticity and resilience, reducing the risk of injuries.

Effective Stretching Techniques:

Dynamic Stretching: Incorporate dynamic stretches (e.g., leg swings, arm circles) into your warm-up routine to prepare muscles for movement and increase blood flow.

Static Stretching: Perform static stretches (e.g., hamstring stretch, quadriceps stretch) after workouts or during cooldowns. Hold each stretch for 15-30 seconds, zeroing in on significant muscle gatherings.

Yoga and Pilates: Participate in yoga or Pilates classes to improve flexibility, balance, and core strength. These practices also emphasize mindfulness and relaxation, supporting overall recovery.

Recovery Strategies:

Rest Days: Schedule regular rest days or active recovery days to allow muscles to repair and rebuild. Light activities such as walking or gentle cycling can enhance blood circulation without taxing muscles.

Hydration: Drink plenty of water throughout the day, especially after workouts, to replenish fluids lost through sweat and support muscle function.

Nutrition: Consume a balanced diet rich in lean proteins, healthy fats, and complex carbohydrates to provide essential nutrients for muscle recovery and energy replenishment.

Foam Rolling: Utilize a froth roller to perform self-myofascial discharge, focusing on close muscles and trigger focuses. This technique can reduce muscle stiffness and improve flexibility.

Sleep: Prioritize adequate sleep to facilitate recovery processes, promote muscle growth, and regulate hormone levels essential for overall health.

Incorporating stretching and recovery practices into your exercise routine enhances the effectiveness of carb cycling by supporting muscle maintenance, preventing injuries, and promoting overall well-being. Adjust your stretching routine based on individual needs and consult with a fitness professional for personalized guidance.

Chapter 9: Lifestyle and Mindset

9.1 Staying Motivated and Consistent

Maintaining motivation and consistency is key to achieving long-term success with carb cycling and any fitness regimen. Here are some effective strategies to stay motivated and consistent:

1. Set Realistic Goals: Establish specific, achievable goals related to your carb cycling journey. Whether it's weight loss, improved fitness levels, or enhanced energy, clear goals provide direction and motivation.

2. Track Your Progress: Keep track of your carb cycling schedule, workouts, and measurements to monitor progress over time. Celebrate achievements, no matter how small, to stay motivated.

3. Create a Routine: Establish a consistent workout schedule and meal plan that fits into your daily life. Consistency breeds habit, making it easier to stick to your carb cycling plan over the long term.

4. Find Enjoyable Activities: Choose exercises and meal options that you enjoy. When you find pleasure in your workouts and meals, you're more likely to stay committed and motivated.

5. Mix It Up: Prevent boredom and plateaus by varying your workouts and meal choices. Try new exercises, recipes, or carb cycling patterns to keep things interesting and challenging.

6. Accountability Partner: Partner with a friend, family member, or a coach who can provide support, encouragement, and accountability. Sharing your goals and progress with someone else can boost motivation.

7. Visualize Success: Picture yourself achieving your goals and visualize the benefits of carb cycling, such as improved health, increased energy, or enhanced fitness. Use visual cues or a vision board to reinforce your motivation.

8. Reward Yourself: Treat yourself to non-food rewards when you reach milestones or achieve goals related to your carb cycling journey.This builds up sure way of behaving and supports proceeded with exertion.

9. Stay Educated: Learn about the benefits of carb cycling and how it aligns with your health and fitness goals. Understanding the science behind the approach can reinforce your commitment.

10. Mindset Matters: Cultivate a positive mindset and resilience. Embrace setbacks as learning opportunities and focus on progress rather than perfection. Consistency over time yields sustainable results.

11. Reflect and Adjust: Regularly assess your progress, challenges, and successes. Adjust your carb cycling plan as needed to ensure it remains effective and aligned with your evolving goals.

By incorporating these strategies into your routine, you can maintain motivation and consistency with carb cycling, leading to long-term success in achieving your health and fitness goals. Adapt these tips to fit your lifestyle and preferences for optimal results.

9.2 Building a Support System

Building a strong support system can significantly enhance your success and motivation in following a carb cycling regimen. Here's how to create and leverage a support network:

1. Family and Friends: Share your goals and reasons for carb cycling with close family members and friends.Their comprehension and consolation can offer profound help and inspiration.

2. Join a Community: Look for online forums, social media groups, or local fitness communities where people share similar goals and experiences with carb cycling. Engage in discussions, seek advice, and celebrate achievements together.

3. Workout Buddies: Find a workout partner or group with whom you can exercise regularly. Having a workout buddy can make workouts more enjoyable, accountable, and motivating.

4. Professional Guidance: Consult with a registered dietitian, nutritionist, or fitness coach who specializes in carb cycling. Their expertise and guidance can ensure you're following a safe and effective plan tailored to your needs.

5. Accountability Partners: Partner with someone who is also committed to their health goals. Check in regularly with each other to share progress, challenges, and provide mutual support.

6. Online Tools and Apps: Use mobile apps or online tools designed for tracking workouts, meals, and progress. Some apps also offer community support features where you can connect with others following similar fitness and nutrition plans.

7. Educational Support: Attend workshops, seminars, or webinars related to carb cycling and nutrition. Learning from experts and connecting with like-minded individuals can deepen your understanding and motivation.

8. Family Involvement: Involve your family in meal planning and preparation. Educate them about carb cycling and its benefits so they can support your dietary choices at home.

9. Celebrate Milestones: Share your achievements, no matter how small, with your support system. Celebrating milestones together reinforces your commitment and encourages continued progress.

10. Be a Supportive Member: Offer encouragement and advice to others in your support network. Being a supportive member of a community fosters positive relationships and reciprocity.

Building a support system can provide encouragement, accountability, and practical advice as you navigate your carb cycling journey. Surround yourself with individuals who understand your goals and are invested in your success, enhancing your motivation and making your health journey more enjoyable and sustainable.

Chapter 10: Long-Term Success

10.1 Transitioning from Weight Loss to Maintenance

Transitioning from weight loss to maintenance phase after achieving your desired goals through carb cycling requires careful planning and adjustments. Here's how to effectively manage this transition:

1. Gradual Adjustments: Gradually increase your daily calorie intake to match your energy expenditure now that you've achieved your weight loss goals. This prevents rapid weight regain while allowing your body to adapt.

2. Monitor Macronutrients: Adjust your carb cycling plan by moderating the frequency or intensity of high and low-carb days based on your new maintenance calorie needs. Focus on maintaining a balanced intake of proteins, healthy fats, and complex carbohydrates.

3. Monitor Your Weight: Regularly monitor your weight and body composition to gauge your progress. Use this feedback to fine-tune your carb cycling approach and ensure you're maintaining your desired weight range.

4. Focus on Nutrient Density: Emphasize nutrient-dense foods to support overall health and energy levels. Include a variety of fruits, vegetables, lean proteins, and whole grains in your diet to meet nutritional needs.

5. Adjust Exercise Routine: Modify your exercise routine to support maintenance goals. Continue with a mix of cardiovascular, strength training, and flexibility exercises to support muscle tone, metabolism, and overall fitness.

6. Mindful Eating: Practice mindful eating habits to prevent overeating and maintain portion control. Pay attention to hunger and satiety cues, and avoid eating out of boredom or emotional triggers.

7. Lifestyle Integration: Integrate healthy eating and physical activity into Center around long haul medical advantages instead of transient outcomes.

8. Celebrate Success: Celebrate your achievements and milestones in weight loss maintenance. Reward yourself with non-food treats or activities that align with your healthy lifestyle.

9. Stay Flexible: Be prepared for fluctuations in weight and adjustments in your carb cycling plan as your body adapts to maintenance mode. Remain adaptable and open to adjusting your methodology on a case by case basis.

10. Seek Support: Continue to seek support from friends, family, or a support group to stay motivated and accountable. Share your maintenance goals and challenges with others who can provide encouragement and guidance.

Transitioning from weight loss to maintenance phase is a significant achievement in your carb cycling journey. By adopting a balanced approach to nutrition, exercise, and lifestyle habits, you can sustain your progress and enjoy long-term health benefits. Adjust your carb cycling plan gradually and stay committed to your overall well-being for continued success.

10.2 Adapting Carb Cycling Over Time

Adapting carb cycling over time is essential for long-term sustainability and continued progress towards your health and fitness goals. Here's how to effectively adjust your carb cycling approach as your needs change:

1. Assess Your Goals: Regularly assess your health and fitness goals to determine if they have evolved. Adjust your carb cycling plan to align with new objectives, whether they involve weight management, athletic performance, or overall health improvement.

2. Evaluate Results: Monitor and evaluate the results of your current carb cycling regimen. Pay attention to how your body responds to different carb intake levels and adjust accordingly based on your progress.

3. Modify Carb Cycling Patterns: Consider modifying the frequency, duration, or intensity of high and low-carb days based on your changing goals and lifestyle. For instance, you may increase high-carb days to support intense workouts or decrease them during periods of reduced activity.

4. Listen to Your Body: Tune into your body's signals and adjust your carb cycling plan accordingly. Pay attention to energy levels, hunger cues, and overall well-being to determine if modifications are needed.

5. Nutrient Timing: Experiment with nutrient timing by adjusting when you consume carbohydrates relative to your workouts or daily activities. Tailor your carb intake to optimize performance, recovery, and energy levels.

6. Seasonal Adjustments: Consider seasonal variations in activity levels and nutritional needs. Adjust your carb cycling plan to accommodate changes in exercise routines, outdoor activities, or dietary preferences during different seasons.

7. Consult with Professionals: Seek guidance from a registered dietitian, nutritionist, or fitness coach when making significant adjustments to your carb cycling plan. Their expertise can help personalize your approach and optimize results.

8. Long-Term Sustainability: Focus on developing sustainable eating habits that support your health and well-being over the long term. Balance carb cycling with a variety of nutrient-dense foods to ensure adequate intake of essential nutrients.

9. Stay Flexible: Remain open to adjusting your carb cycling plan as needed. Be patient with yourself and allow time for your body to adapt to new dietary patterns and fitness routines.

10. Track Progress: Continuously track your progress, including changes in weight, body composition, performance metrics, and overall well-being. Use this information to refine your carb cycling strategy and maintain motivation.

Adapting carb cycling over time involves a balance of monitoring your body's responses, adjusting to new goals, and maintaining a flexible approach to nutrition and fitness. By staying mindful of your needs and making informed adjustments, you can sustainably optimize your health and fitness journey with carb cycling.

10.3 Celebrating Milestones and Successes

Celebrating milestones and successes along your carb cycling journey is crucial for maintaining motivation and reinforcing positive behaviors. Here's why and how to celebrate your achievements:

1. Recognition of Progress: Celebrating milestones allows you to acknowledge your hard work and dedication. It reinforces the positive changes you've made in your health, fitness, and overall well-being through carb cycling.

2. Boost in Motivation: Recognizing and celebrating your successes can boost motivation to continue pursuing your goals. It provides a sense of accomplishment and encourages you to stay committed to your carb cycling plan.

3. Positive Reinforcement: Celebrating milestones acts as positive reinforcement for sticking to healthy habits. It reinforces the idea that your efforts are worthwhile and encourages continued adherence to your nutrition and fitness regimen.

4. Reflection and Gratitude: Taking time to celebrate milestones allows for reflection on your journey and the obstacles you've overcome. It fosters gratitude for the progress made and the support received from others.

5. Maintaining Momentum: Celebrating successes helps maintain momentum in your carb cycling journey. It encourages a positive mindset and reinforces your commitment to long-term health and fitness goals.

How to Celebrate Milestones:
- Set Milestone Goals: Break down your larger goals into smaller milestones (e.g., weight loss milestones, fitness achievements) that are achievable and measurable.

- Reward Yourself: Treat yourself to non-food rewards when you achieve milestones. Consider activities you enjoy, such as buying new workout gear, booking a massage, or enjoying a relaxing day off.

- Share Your Achievements: Share your successes with friends, family, or a support group. Celebrate with loved ones who have supported you on your journey and acknowledge their role in your success.

- Reflect and Plan Ahead: Take time to reflect on what you've accomplished and how far you've come. Use this reflection to set new goals and continue progressing in your carb cycling and overall health journey.

- Create Rituals: Establish rituals or traditions around celebrating milestones, such as writing in a journal, creating a vision board, or taking progress photos to document your achievements.

By celebrating milestones and successes, you reinforce positive behaviors, maintain motivation, and foster a sense of accomplishment in your carb cycling journey. Embrace each milestone as a stepping stone towards your long-term health and fitness goals, and continue to celebrate your progress along the way.

Chapter 11: Conclusion

11.1 Final Thoughts

As you conclude your exploration of carb cycling for women over 50, it's important to reflect on the journey and consider these final thoughts:

Personalized Approach: Carb cycling is a versatile approach that can be tailored to individual preferences, health goals, and lifestyles. Experiment with different cycling patterns and adjust based on what works best for you.

Long-Term Sustainability: Focus on adopting sustainable habits that promote overall health and well-being. Embrace carb cycling as part of a balanced lifestyle that includes nutrient-dense foods, regular exercise, and adequate rest.

Continuous Learning: Stay informed about nutrition, fitness trends, and scientific research related to carb cycling. Education empowers you to make informed decisions and adapt your approach over time.

Celebrating Successes: Recognize and celebrate your achievements, no matter how small. Milestones and successes provide motivation and reinforce positive behaviors that contribute to your overall health journey.

Support Network: Surround yourself with a supportive network of friends, family, or online communities who share similar health goals. Their encouragement and accountability can enhance your motivation and success.

Mind-Body Connection: Listen to your body's signals and adjust your carb cycling plan accordingly. Practice mindful eating, prioritize self-care, and maintain a positive mindset throughout your journey.

Setting New Goals: Use your carb cycling experience as a foundation for setting new goals and continuing to improve your health and fitness. Whether it's maintaining weight, building muscle, or improving endurance, set clear, achievable goals to strive towards.

Seeking Professional Guidance: Consult with healthcare professionals, such as registered dietitians or fitness coaches, for personalized advice and support. Their expertise can help optimize your carb cycling plan and ensure it aligns with your health needs.

Enjoying the Process: Embrace the journey towards better health and enjoy the benefits of carb cycling. Stay flexible, patient with yourself, and adaptable to changes as you navigate through different phases of your health and fitness goals.

By integrating these final thoughts into your approach to carb cycling, you can maximize its benefits and sustain your progress over the long term. Embrace the journey as an opportunity for growth, self-discovery, and improved well-being.